A Guide for Lewy Body Dementia Caregivers

I0121101

A Guide for Lewy Body Dementia Caregivers: Caring with Compassion is a daughter's heartbreaking yet hopeful account of her secondary caregiving journey for her mother who has Lewy body dementia (LBD).

This compassion guidebook is a friendly and practical companion for helping those affected by LBD and other memory-related diseases. The author offers guidance about coping with the strain of being a caregiver and the importance of self-compassion as well as compassion, whilst on the journey. She uses her personal experience to touch on relatable subjects associated with memory loss such as object misplacement, visual changes, family gatherings, hospital visits, respite care, memory care and anticipatory grief. This book includes an introductory chapter on the science behind LBD by an internationally renowned behavioral neurologist. It discusses the core symptoms and latest research to ground the personal experiences in science. Each following chapter contains a lesson learned and is a bite-sized length, so busy caregivers can read as time allows.

This is essential reading for those caring for someone with LBD to help understand the realities of this disease and to support them along the way.

Kimberly Pellicore is an established writer and editor. She is a graduate of Texas A&M University and finds her words shine brightest when she is using them to help others. She is a proud wife and mother of two who lives in Houston, Texas.

Dr. Bruce L. Miller holds the A.W. and Mary Margaret Clausen Distinguished Professorship in Neurology at UC San Francisco and is the founding director of the Memory and Aging Center and the Global Brain Health Institute. As a behavioral neurologist, he studies social behavior, creativity and disorders of the aging brain.

A Guide for Lewy Body Dementia Caregivers

Caring with Compassion

Kimberly Pellicore with
Bruce L. Miller

Routledge
Taylor & Francis Group

NEW YORK AND LONDON

Designed cover image: Cover image created by Selah Sweet
and reproduced with permission

First published 2026
by Routledge
605 Third Avenue, New York, NY 10158

and by Routledge
4 Park Square, Milton Park, Abingdon, Oxon, OX14 4RN

Routledge is an imprint of the Taylor & Francis Group, an informa business

ISBN: 9781041108009 (hbk)
ISBN: 9781041107958 (pbk)
ISBN: 9781003656890 (ebk)

DOI: 10.4324/9781003656890

Typeset in Sabon
by codeMantra

Dedication

For my mom, who is one of the strongest women I have ever known. You are a beloved daughter, sister, wife, mother, grandmother and friend. Your love and strength are things of legend, and I will do my best to continue that tradition. I am forever proud to be your daughter. Thanks for being my mom. I love you, always.

Contents

Foreword

The compassion guidebook you are holding in your hand is a friendly and practical companion for helping those affected by Lewy body dementia (LBD) and other memory-related diseases. Kimberly Pellicore offers a "how to manual" through documenting her deeply personal experiences in such an engaging style that you can't help but feel less afraid and less alone.

I have deep admiration for Kimberly to have written this book, which is something I never could have done for two reasons. First, because I was the primary caregiver for my belated husband Robin Williams. It would not have been physically, mentally or emotionally possible for me to write this at the time. And second, we did not have an accurate diagnosis for what Robin was suffering from until after his death. It was only revealed in autopsy that Robin had diffuse Lewy body disease. If we'd had the name of the disease while Robin was alive rather than being on a diagnostic odyssey, this book would have been tremendously helpful.

Kimberly writes from her perspective as a secondary caregiver, a daughter helping her dad care for her mom. She is armed with her mom's diagnosis of Lewy body dementia. This book is filled with Kimberly's experience and discoveries, a travel companion if you will, to help as you go down the road of caring for someone with LBD. It contains research along with charming self-observations and honest self-assessments. Her compassionate voice shines through her many insights providing a heartwarming bridge for the reader to understand the realities of this disease.

This book can be helpful not only for those affected by LBD but also for those affected by other memory diseases. As Kimberly points out, it is not uncommon for someone to have a few things going on. Robin, in fact, not only had LBD but also Parkinson's plus the amyloid plaques and tau tangles of Alzheimer's disease. This guidebook provides just that – guidance, what to expect and tips to help along the way if you have a loved one with these diseases.

There is also a third reason I couldn't have written this book. LBD can be brutal. There's no easy way of saying that. It takes a special individual to be able to go through this experience, research it in real time and share those discoveries with others. It takes courage and emotional fortitude.

Like Kimberly, I dove into the research, making it a full-time job. I found it emotionally easier after my husband's passing to focus on the science. My heart felt like a wasteland after the experience, and I'm quite sure if someone floated the idea to me of writing a guidebook at the time I would have just involuntarily thrown up! What I could do though was research the science behind the disease and try my best to share our experience and raise awareness and funds for LBD research.

Kimberly's faith is evident, and I appreciate her openness in sharing that. I too had and have a faith that has gotten me through the storms in life and been a companion during the good times and the bad. It's been my rock. The LBD experience stretched my muscles of faith. My prayer for you is that whatever faith muscles you already have, may they grow stronger and more flexible with your experiences in life, including if you are having an LBD experience.

I expect this book will prove to be a steadfast companion for you no matter where you are on your journey.

Susan Schneider Williams
Susan is a professional fine artist and advocate. She has become a prominent voice for brain disease research and awareness since her husband Robin Williams's passing in 2014 from LBD. To learn more about Susan's work, please visit ssfineart.com.

Preface

I look at the woman in the bathroom mirror. At first, I do not recognize her. She looks older and several pounds heavier than she did just five short years ago. Shadows haunt her pale features like maybe she hasn't had enough sleep. She does have makeup on, but even it cannot disguise the invisible scars of heartbreak. I don't know this woman looking back at me, but I feel compelled to hug her.

Minutes pass as I stand with a fixed stare into the mirror. There is something else about her that I just can't put my finger on. Several more minutes pass as I hold the woman's gaze and then suddenly, I see it. The thing that gave me pause, that I couldn't put my finger on, is not her external appearance at all. It is the steady strength that radiates from within her.

It is quiet and unassuming. It does not beg to be seen or to be given a microphone or a stage. It is hard earned. It is laced with heartache and hope. It is resolute. It does not abhor tears and does not shy away from the heaviness in her heart, for that is where her strength is forged.

I realize with a touch of pride, that the woman in the mirror really is me. I am not the same person I was before this journey began, but, by God's grace, I am learning to appreciate the person I have become and what the journey has taught me.

I am tired but I am wiser. I am heartbroken but I am hopeful. I am sad but I am grateful. I am a work in progress and will be until God calls me home.

Yet, amidst all the changes, one thing remains. I will *always* be my mother's daughter, and she will *always* be Mom to me.

I originally wrote this about myself, wondering if other caregivers of loved ones with Lewy body dementia (LBD) might see themselves in it too. However, when I finished writing this, I was struck at how many of these very same words could have just as easily been written by my mom, perhaps the last time she was able to recognize her own reflection.

LBD is a ruthless disease. Really, ruthless is too nice of a word. I don't think they make a word that accurately encompasses the hell that this diagnosis can be for the person who is diagnosed or their caregivers.

But...

I pray, despite all the disease took from her and continues to take today, that she sees past the changes in her outward appearance to the overwhelming strength that quietly lies underneath. If you love someone who is in the middle to late stages of LBD, or another memory-based disease, then you may be asking, "Amidst all the chaos, the hallucinations and the paranoia of the diagnosed, how are they displaying strength?"

Consider this. What would you call the trait that a person with this disease displays when they pull themselves up by the bootstraps every single day to face another 24 hours of confusion, sadness, anger and pain? Oh...and then repeat this process daily as they continue to deteriorate.

If that is not a picture of strength, I am not sure what is. Honestly, it exhausts me watching it from the outside. I simply cannot imagine what it is like to have to embrace and live that madness personally each day.

My mom's strength may look like happy laughter in her sleep. It may look like getting completely dressed by herself. It may look like having unintelligible conversations with imaginary people. It may look like crying on a bad day. It may look like anger at the disease. What it is not, however, is giving up.

Even as her journey appears to be drawing nearer to a close, she is still teaching me, and I am taking every single lesson to heart.

My prayer is that what I have learned will strengthen the resolve of caregivers as well as that of family and friends who love someone with LBD or a related memory disease. We are in this together. You are not alone.

Acknowledgments

Mom, you are the most courageous woman I have ever known. You are powerfully changing lives through the story you bravely live out day after day. Thank you for giving me the strength to tell it.

Dad, I am incredibly proud to be your daughter. You have loved mom well for more than half a century and have taught me the art of loving someone with all that you have, every single day. Even when battling cancer, you never stopped being a phenomenal caregiver.

The thing about being part of the sandwich generation as a caregiver is that it impacts the whole family. To my husband, Mark, thank you for standing by my side and helping things continue to run smoothly at home when caregiving calls me away. Tyler and Maggie, thank you for your patience and understanding as I continue to learn how to balance being a caregiver and mom. Your hugs and laughter buoy me in ways you may never fully know. You are my people and there is no one I would rather do life with.

Tiffany Woolf, I might never have connected with Susan had it not been for your heart for storytelling. This book is possible because you took a leap of faith on my behalf. Thank you!

Susan Schneider Williams, you are a blessing to the Lewy body dementia community and to me personally. There are no words to adequately thank you for opening your heart, championing my work and reliving parts of your journey with Robin as you read my own. Your dedication to advocating for awareness, education and research of this disease is inspiring. You lead with understanding, compassion and grace and undoubtedly honor Robin's memory by helping others. I am grateful to know you and blessed to call you friend.

To Dr. Miller, I am beyond honored to have you be a supporting author for this work. You have believed in my words since the beginning and have continued to be a great source of encouragement along the way. This book would not have been complete without your chapter detailing the science of Lewy body dementia. Thank you for all of the many ways you serve.

To my team at Taylor & Francis Group, I could not have done this without you. Thank you for giving heartfelt stories like mine a home. Lucy Kennedy, thank you for tirelessly advocating for my work. Simran Kaur, thank for your patience every step of the way.

There is a giant chasm between putting words to paper and having the confidence to share them with the world. I can say with absolute certainty that my story would still be unfinished and still buried in the recesses of my computer without some very persistent cheerleaders. To Kelly Guzman, you are an angel for making me promise to keep writing and believe in myself. To Quinn Kelly, thank you for listening and inspiring me to share in the midst of the journey. To Helen Ditges, I am grateful for your marketing wisdom.

A special thanks also goes to Amanda Prieto for looking after my words; Selah Sweet for painting my book cover artwork; Dr. Burt Palmer, Nancy Russell, Laura De La Rosa, Susan Tibbetts, Betty Jo Frindell, Tonya Johnston, Nikki Smith, Kelli Elkins, Shawna Fritsch, Genell Pippett, the ladies of Grace and countless others for being sounding boards and encouragers.

Lastly, and perhaps most importantly, I thank my Lord and Savior, Jesus Christ. Without you, this story would not have hope. Without you knitting together the pieces of heartbreak and tears for good, there would be no book to be a resource for others. You continue to be my rock, my fortress and my deliverer (Psalm 118). To God be the glory.

Part 1

The Science

Bruce L. Miller

Chapter 1

What Is Lewy Body Dementia?

What Is Dementia with Lewy Bodies?

Dementia with Lewy bodies (DLB) is a brain disorder that can cause problems with thinking, sleep, movement, mood and behavior. It is caused by abnormal clumps of a protein called *alpha-synuclein* that accumulate in brain cells. These clumps are called "Lewy bodies." They cause brain cells to stop working correctly and eventually die. What causes these changes in the brain is not yet fully understood. DLB comprises up to 24% of all neurodegenerative dementia cases, making it the second most prevalent neurodegenerative dementia, only exceeded by Alzheimer's disease (AD) (Figure 1.1).

Although typically beginning at age 50 or above, younger people may sometimes develop the disease. DLB is a progressive disease, meaning symptoms start slowly and worsen over time. Symptoms vary from person to person, but the disease can begin with hallucinations, depression or anxiety, disordered sleep, constipation or sexual dysfunction or slowing of movement. These symptoms are broadly classified into cognitive, movement, autonomic and psychiatric.

DLB is characterized by dementia in combination with core clinical features of rapid eye movement (REM) behavior disorder (RBD), parkinsonism, cognitive and alertness fluctuations and visual hallucinations. In addition, several supportive clinical features, indicative biomarkers and supportive biomarkers help establish a clinical diagnosis.

Table 1.1 highlights the diagnostic criteria of DLB.

DOI: 10.4324/9781003656890-2

Typical Brain

Dementia with Lewy Bodies

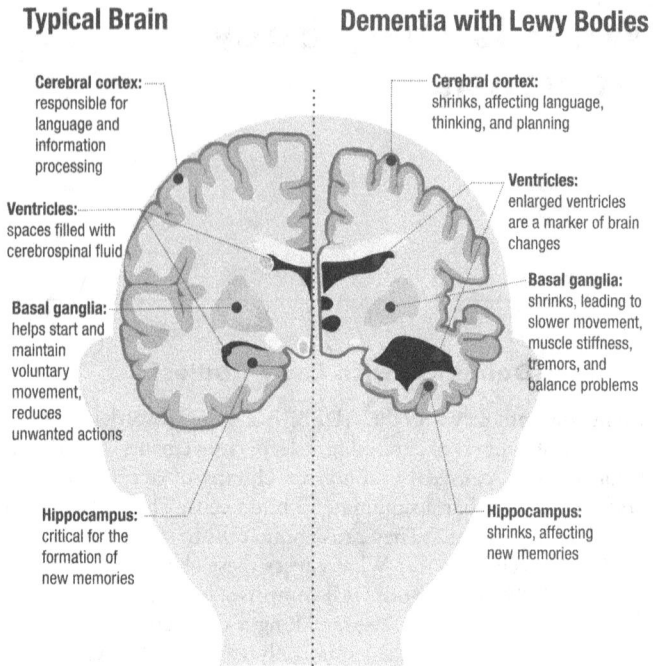

Cerebral cortex: responsible for language and information processing

Ventricles: spaces filled with cerebrospinal fluid

Basal ganglia: helps start and maintain voluntary movement, reduces unwanted actions

Hippocampus: critical for the formation of new memories

Cerebral cortex: shrinks, affecting language, thinking, and planning

Ventricles: enlarged ventricles are a marker of brain changes

Basal ganglia: shrinks, leading to slower movement, muscle stiffness, tremors, and balance problems

Hippocampus: shrinks, affecting new memories

Figure 1.1 Areas of the brain affected by DLB.

Cognitive Symptoms

Problems with Executive Function

Executive dysfunction manifests as difficulty with multitasking, such as listening to music while organizing files or taking notes while listening to a lecture. They may also have trouble with problem-solving, such as managing a budget effectively. Often, people with impaired executive function are unable to break down a problem into manageable steps or create a clear plan of action. They may have difficulty navigating social situations, such as resolving a conflict with a friend or colleague, due to the inability to clearly articulate their thoughts and consider different perspectives or due to making impulsive

Table 1.1 Diagnostic Criteria for DLB

Dementia	Cognitive decline in more than one cognitive domain, significant enough to affect functional abilities. Declines in memory, attention, executive cognitive function and visuospatial abilities are common.
Core clinical features	• Fluctuating cognition, attention and alertness • Recurrent visual hallucinations • REM Sleep Behavior Disorder (RBD) • Parkinsonism (one or more spontaneous features, such as slowness of movement, rest tremor or rigidity)
Indicative biomarkers	• Reduced dopamine transporter uptake in the basal ganglia • Low uptake on ^{123}I-metaiodobenzylguanidine (MIBG) myocardial scintigraphy • Sleep study evidence of REM sleep without the temporary muscular immobility (atonia)
Probable DLB diagnosis	Two or more core clinical features, with or without an indicative biomarker OR One core clinical feature, plus one or more indicative biomarkers

comments in a conversation without thinking through the potential consequences.

Problems with Visual-Spatial Tasks

Patients may misjudge a distance or depth as well as misidentify objects. They may struggle to navigate a familiar environment and get lost easily, even in places they've been many times before, due to difficulty judging distances and spatial orientation. Additionally, they may not be able to accurately park their car or find the correct aisle in a grocery store. Frequent car accidents may reflect this spatial difficulty. Another indication of impaired visuospatial function may be bumping into objects frequently due to misjudging their position in space.

Impaired Concentration or Attention

This symptom may manifest as someone who frequently loses focus mid-conversation, struggles to follow instructions, exhibits difficulty completing tasks due to distractions, fluctuates unpredictably in alertness throughout the day, stares into space for extended periods and shows difficulty staying engaged in activities that require sustained attention, even for short durations. Sometimes, they may appear "zoned out" or mentally absent even while seemingly awake. Due to this problem with attention, people may forget what they were planning to do when they walk from one room to another or stop mid-sentence while losing track of their thoughts.

Memory Deficits

Unlike AD, memory loss may not be the most prominent feature in the early stages of the disease, but this often appears as the disease progresses and can fluctuate significantly. As with attention, a patient may experience periods of good memory followed by noticeable memory loss. The other cognitive issues, like visual-spatial problems and attention difficulties, may be more prominent early on.

Treatment of Cognitive Symptoms

Cholinesterase inhibitors are first-line therapy to improve cognition in people with DLB, including improvements in memory, attention and global cognitive measures. Rivastigmine and donepezil have been studied extensively in people with DLB, with a high level of evidence supporting treatment. As a class, cholinesterase inhibitors may cause mild to moderate side effects (in 15%– 20% of people) that may include nausea, anorexia, diarrhea, rhinorrhea, vivid dreams and, rarely, muscle cramps, bradycardia or syncope.

Memantine, an NMDA (N-methyl-D-aspartate) receptor modulator, is a second-line medication for DLB. It can improve measures of attention and episodic recognition memory in people with DLB. Memantine has a good side-effect profile but can cause dizziness or confusion (e.g., reports of feeling detached or "spacey") in some people. It can be added to a cholinesterase inhibitor, especially in people with mild to moderate dementia symptoms.

Motor Features

Motor symptoms in DLB resemble those of Parkinson's disease and are referred to as parkinsonism. Parkinsonism affects up to 85% of people with DLB, preceding or sometimes following memory and cognitive symptoms. These movement-related issues occur because Lewy bodies affect the basal ganglia in the brain, which are involved in motor control and coordination. People with DLB may experience difficulties with:

- Slowness of movement (bradykinesia).
- Muscle stiffness (rigidity).
- Tremors (shaking).
- Balance (postural instability).

In the early stages of DLB, motor symptoms may be mild and overlooked. As the disease progresses, movement problems become more noticeable and can interfere with daily activities. Like Parkinson's disease, the severity of motor issues in DLB varies across individuals. One of the most troubling aspects of motor symptoms in DLB is their unpredictability. A person may move relatively well one day and struggle significantly the next. This fluctuation can be frustrating for both patients and caregivers.

Although there is no cure, various therapies and strategies can help improve movement:

1 Physical and occupational therapy guided by professionals.
2 Exercise programs to maintain strength and flexibility by encouraging large, deliberate movements. Chair exercises may be helpful for those with severe movement limitations.

3 Using assistive devices, like canes and walkers, to prevent falls. Button hooks, adaptive clothing and Velcro shoes can make dressing easier.

4 Creating a fall-proof environment at home by removing rugs or other trip hazards, installing grab bars and improving the lighting conditions.

5 Medications (carefully balanced by a doctor based on each person's symptoms) may include Levodopa (L-DOPA) or dopamine agonists. They are short-acting but help increase the dopamine levels in the basal ganglia.

Autonomic Symptoms

The autonomic nervous system controls involuntary bodily functions, such as heart rate, digestion, blood pressure, temperature regulation and control of bowel movements, urination and sexual function. In DLB, Lewy bodies deposit in the brain stem and autonomic nervous system and disrupt communication, leading to autonomic dysfunction in about 60%–80% of patients. Common autonomic symptoms in DLB include:

- Low blood pressure (orthostatic hypotension).
- Urinary urgency or incontinence (difficulty controlling the bladder).
- Constipation.
- Sexual dysfunction (reduced libido or difficulty with erection and orgasm).
- Excessive salivation (drooling) or dry mouth.
- Temperature regulation problems (sweating too much or too little, feeling too hot or too cold).

Autonomic dysfunction can significantly impact daily activities. For example, dizziness from low blood pressure makes it challenging to move around safely. Bladder problems may cause embarrassment or lead to frequent trips to the bathroom, and constipation can cause significant discomfort. Caregivers often need to monitor these symptoms and adjust daily routines to help manage them.

Other interventions that may help include standing up slowly and drinking more fluids to help prevent drops in blood pressure. A doctor may also prescribe compression stockings or medications like Midodrine and Fludrocortisone. For bladder problems, scheduling bathroom trips and reducing fluids before bedtime can reduce accidents. Medications may help control incontinence. For constipation, a high-fiber diet, hydration and regular movement can help. Dressing in layers and avoiding extreme temperatures can help manage discomfort and regulate temperature.

Neuropsychiatric Symptoms

DLB affects not only those who live with it but also their loved ones who care for and support them. The disease transforms how a person thinks, feels and behaves. Understanding these symptoms allows us to navigate this journey with patience, empathy and the necessary tools to face daily challenges.

Clarity and Confusion

Imagine being fully alert and focused one minute, only to suddenly feel disoriented or overwhelmingly drowsy in the next. Many people with DLB experience these swings. Their ability to pay attention and concentrate can fluctuate from hour to hour or day to day, making it difficult to predict what will happen next. It is essential to understand that these changes are part of the disease, not something they can control.

Seeing What Isn't There (Hallucinations)

Visual hallucinations are common in DLB. A loved one may describe seeing people, animals or objects that aren't there. These visions can be vivid and detailed, sometimes comforting and other times unsettling. If this happens, stay calm and provide gentle reassurance without arguing about what may or may not be real. Your steadiness has the potential to be an anchor amid your loved one's confusion.

Unshakable Beliefs (Delusions)

Delusions are strong beliefs that are not based in reality. Someone with DLB may believe they are being robbed or that an impostor has taken a family member's place. It can be very distressing for the individual having these thoughts, as well as their caregivers. Rather than challenge the belief, acknowledge the emotion they are experiencing, validating their feelings, even if you do not share their perception. Delusions in DLB, like many clinical features of this disorder, may fluctuate and sometimes disappear for many weeks.

Emotional Changes

Mood fluctuations are an essential feature of DLB. Your loved one may feel sad, anxious or no longer connected to things they used to enjoy. It hurts to see them lose interest in things they love or to seem removed from reality. But these changes are not personal; they are a manifestation of the disease. Simply being there, providing little acts of affection or simply accompanying them can make a big difference. Severe depression is quite common with DLB and, when accompanied by psychosis, can be life-threatening. With depression, these patients may blame themselves for family or world conflicts, and suicidality tends to occur. Treatment should be referred to psychiatrists with expertise in elderly care, as they may require both antidepressants and antipsychotics.

Restless Nights and Sleep Disturbances

Sleep disorders are common in DLB. Some people may physically act out their dreams, which can be dangerous as they might shout, move abruptly or even fall out of bed, unintentionally injuring themselves or their bed partner. This behavior is called RBD and can precede the onset of other symptoms related to DLB by many years. In some cases, the sleep disorder occurs after the onset of symptoms. Another sleep-related symptom common in DLB is excessive sleepiness. During the daytime, many patients feel excessively sleepy despite sleeping at night. Establishing a relaxing bedtime routine and a safe sleeping environment can help alleviate these issues.

Caring with Compassion

Dealing with challenging behaviors can be overwhelming. Remember that these behaviors are not intentional; they are symptoms of DLB. While managing these symptoms is essential, caregiver support is equally critical, as the challenges of DLB can be physically and emotionally exhausting. Caregivers need time to recharge, so rest, short breaks and respite care are vital to reducing stress and preventing burnout. Ensuring caregivers receive adequate support benefits their well-being and enhances the quality of care they provide.

Part 2

The Experience

Kimberly Pellicore

Chapter 2

The Brain Can Be as Beautiful as It Is Dangerous

Until my mom's Lewy body dementia (LBD) diagnosis, I had not experienced being around someone with a memory disease and honestly had no idea how powerful and dangerous the brain can be. The average adult brain is estimated to weigh just three pounds, yet the fact that it controls what happens within the other 100–200+ pounds of body weight makes it a force to be reckoned with.

I am amazed at how many things this little three-pound organ controls within the body. It is both awesome and scary that something that small can wield so much power. Keeping this in mind, it is not a stretch to realize that when memory disease or dementia compromises part of the brain, the effects can be profound.

As I write this and to my knowledge, there are still no definitive, gold-standard tests comprehensive enough to diagnose LBD with absolute certainty while a person is still living. This presents a challenge for both the doctor and the patient.

For my mom, the diagnosis was a complicated journey that incorporated a combination of patient history, medical testing and neuropsychological tests.

In the beginning, there seemed to be only small changes, such as my mom having trouble remembering a date or time, something that was highly unusual for her. She used to be the most organized person I knew. After a hard conversation followed by my gentle prodding, my mom quite grudgingly agreed to mention it to her general practitioner at her upcoming appointment.

After some initial testing by my mom's primary care physician, there was a consensus that the issue at play could be as simple as a vitamin shortage, specifically B12. After a couple of

DOI: 10.4324/9781003656890-4

vitamin shots, we were already noticing some improvement and felt a huge sense of relief.

However, in a matter of months, any initial improvements we saw in my mom soon regressed. Although she now had what the doctor believed to be an adequate amount of B12 in her system, suddenly in the isolation of COVID-19 my mom forgot how to perform relatively simple tasks like taking her medication and operating her smartphone. Even worse, my mom was unable to recognize who her husband and family were.

After an MRI that basically came up clean, my mom's neurologist sent her to a special testing center for conversational and cognitive exams. This simple but comprehensive testing lasted for hours, most likely in an effort to test her cognitive endurance. Unfortunately, she became so agitated during the exams, she refused to cooperate and requested to stop. She reluctantly agreed to come back again to finish the testing. My mom taught college-level courses at one time, so I believe that normally she would be able to complete the testing without issue. I think she still had enough cognitive bandwidth at the time of testing to know there was something wrong if she was unable to do so.

After a professional evaluation of her testing results, the facilitators called with what they believed to be the most accurate diagnosis given her physician's and neurologist's findings, LBD.

I like knowing what I am up against rather than fighting the unknown, so I threw myself into research. It turned out there was not much helpful guidance to be had other than that LBD diagnoses were still relatively uncommon, and everyone seemed to respond differently to the disease.

Everything my mom experienced early on seemed highly advanced for a new LBD diagnosis. Now, years into this journey, I am hearing more and more about people who have LBD, Alzheimer's and Parkinson's diagnoses simultaneously. It may be that my mom is dealing with more than just the one diagnosis, but we likely will not know conclusively until she passes.

I would be remiss to end this chapter about the power of the brain without talking about what a person with LBD donating their brain to science may be able to do for others. The answer is that it may provide researchers with much needed answers.

This was something my mom felt strongly about. She wanted to donate her brain to research if there was a chance it could prevent someone else from experiencing the hell she had.

Should your loved one choose to donate their brain to a specific field of study such as memory disease, it is important to act now as the process requires advanced planning. Find the right organization for you, fill out the forms and get familiar with the protocol that must be followed before and after your loved one passes. This is critical to the integrity of the organ for it to be professionally studied.

Our loved ones struggling with memory disease may find their brains do not work quite the same way anymore, but we, as their caregivers, can learn from them so their suffering is not in vain. We can begin pledging to take better care of our brains now. If you are not sure where to start, I recommend Hilarity for Charity's HFC Universe program which can be accessed through their website.

Chapter 3

Control Is Only an Illusion

Right, wrong or indifferent, I am a fixer. I used to think that to be this way was both admirable and innocent. While it can still be admirable, I no longer see it as completely innocent. In fact, I see it as more of a nod to my need for control than an inherently altruistic motivation. It has only taken me 47 years to embrace this little nugget of truth.

In my opinion, being diagnosed with a memory disease or loving someone with a memory disease is to acknowledge that you do not have control. And find out it is possible that you never did. However, this tends to be more of a gradual realization.

For example, currently we cannot control if a disease like Lewy body dementia (LBD) develops inside the brain. However, there are steps we can take to practice good brain health and take better care of the body. Yet, we must still acknowledge that even these efforts may only delay the inevitable. It should not negate us practicing better brain health, but it helps to adjust our expectations accordingly.

Loss of control over a diagnosis was something I did not like nor understand, yet I accepted it. But not anything beyond that.

Diagnosis in hand, I sought all the information I could about LBD. Although being well informed about a diagnosis is recommended, I tend to take that sentiment to the extreme. This is because having all the information can feel like having control. Yet, it is not. Ask me how I know.

For months and months, I researched my mom's diagnosis like it was my job. At the time, there was not an abundance of information available. This usually had me running in circles and chasing links and resources that led to the black hole that surfing

DOI: 10.4324/9781003656890-5

online usually does. What it did not get me was any closer to knowing what to expect.

I did not have a clear idea of what stage of the disease my mom was in. I did not have much information about treatment. I knew no one with this diagnosis or anyone who had a loved one with this diagnosis. There were no comparisons or contrasts to be made.

Rather than accept defeat, I put together a binder containing contact information for my mom's physicians, medications she was currently on and any articles that offered helpful tips. Then I made three copies of the binder: one for me, one for my dad and one for my sister. These were beneficial actions to take, but my motivation was the act of being busy – my antidote to loss of control.

I will never forget the immense effort I put into the creation of those binders in hopes it would help us keep up with important information and then continuously add to it. My parents had come over that morning and I had my dad's binder sitting out on the kitchen table. Within ten minutes of them arriving, I could not find that binder anywhere. My mom had "moved" it, and it could not be found.

From that point forward, loss of control reigned. My teens were at home learning virtually during the pandemic, and I was trying to ensure they were all set while at the same time working from home myself and helping my parents. There would be hours where joy and routine almost seemed within reach, but then I would get a call from my mom or dad that changed everything on a dime.

Even though my mom is in a good memory care facility today and I see her often, those phone calls sometimes still come. A few months ago, my daughter and I went wedding dress shopping for a friend's daughter. It was a beautiful day of shopping, lunching and daydreaming. I distinctly remember talking with my daughter about how much fun the day had been as we were driving to the second wedding dress shop. Upon arrival at the store, I received a call from my dad that mom was suddenly not doing well. And just like that, the proverbial other shoe dropped.

Sometimes it still feels as though I live my life just waiting for the other shoe to drop. The temptation to enjoy a wonderful day or great news is always interrupted by a little voice in the back of my head urging me not to be too happy, or bad news might swoop in and ruin everything. This really is no way to live life. It is something I am working on.

One of the worst parts about grasping for control the way you grab to catch something breakable before it hits the ground is that we are not the only people it hurts. Sometimes it hurts those we love who are experiencing memory loss.

During the years since mom's diagnosis, we have found and spent time with a handful of other families who also had a loved one with a memory disease. These families were all at different stages of acceptance and grief. One day I saw a man desperate to have a normal meal with his wife at the memory care home. He worked for more than 20 minutes to get her from sitting in a wheelchair to sitting in a regular dining chair. From my point of view, he was trying to help, honor her and retain some sense of normalcy. Yet, there was probably a little bit of a need for control operating in there too. Unfortunately, at the end of their struggle, the wife appeared significantly agitated and emotional...and still in her wheelchair. It struck me as so sad that all his work to control dinner only resulted in him and his wife becoming beyond frustrated.

I share this without too much judgment because I know there have been multiple times when I have inadvertently done something similar. I can almost guarantee you that along the way I have made choices I thought were for my mom, but perhaps best served me. Sometimes the need for control can blind us in the moment, but hindsight can help us see it for what it is.

For most people, truly accepting a loss of control is not something that happens overnight. And that is okay. However, if you are lucky enough to figure it out, do us all a favor and please share.

Until then, I have come to believe that there is immense power in relinquishing control. It may cost those of us who have controlling tendencies in the beginning, but the freedom it gives way to will be well worth the sacrifice – for ourselves and the people we are caring for.

Chapter 4

To Be Scared Is Okay,
to Be Absent Is Not

To watch a loved one walk through Lewy body dementia (LBD) (or any memory loss disease) is scary. I say this because I think there is power in acknowledging it upfront. Yes, this journey can be frightening for both patient and caregiver, but with a diagnosis comes at least a starting point for facing whatever lies ahead.

To our knowledge, no one in our family has ever been diagnosed with LBD. All I knew about the disease at the time of mom's diagnosis was that Robin Williams had been posthumously diagnosed with it. In other words, I knew next to nothing about what to expect.

This was a problem because, for me personally, the unknown is scarier than knowing what I am actually up against.

I didn't know mom would forget who her family was before a diagnosis ever came and that it would breed distrust.
I didn't know mom's brain would make her see disturbing people and images that were not really there.
I didn't know mom would think my dad was at least two different people, neither of which she thought to be her husband.
I didn't know mom would forget that her house of more than thirty years was her home.
I didn't know my mom would become so scared about not knowing us as family, that she would call the police.
I didn't know I would get calls all hours of the night with her being scared about the other people living in her house (there was no one there but my dad).

DOI: 10.4324/9781003656890-6

I didn't know how hard this would be on my dad's mental, emotional and physical health.

I didn't know. I didn't know. I didn't know. What I didn't know about LBD and how it would affect my mom could fill the earth ten times over. It. Was. Terrifying.

Yet...

I figured I had two choices as a daughter helping her dad care for her mom. I could let my fear keep me from spending precious time with my hurting mom (and dad) in the name of self-preservation, or I could suck it up and love my mom through all her own fears just like she did for me growing up. There was no question, the latter was my final decision.

I guess some people would say when it came to helping my mom and dad navigate LBD, I was "doing it scared." And you know what? That is okay because I did it anyway. I was present to hold mom in my arms when she sobbed over the brutality of this insidious disease. I was there to watch and spend time with her so my dad could have a mental break. I took mom to get her hair done. I took mom to shop at small local stores. I answered the phone in the wee hours when dad needed me to confirm to mom that the man holding the phone up to her ear was indeed her husband and my dad. It was heart wrenching, but I would do it all again in a heartbeat.

It is important to remember I was a secondary caregiver that was able to pop in and help whenever I could, but then I got to go home to my family, my house and my routine. The main caregiver, in this case my dad, did not have this luxury. He took care of my mom around the clock and probably endured most of what I write about feeling in this book times 20. If you are a primary caregiver, please do not forget to take care of yourself. If you are a secondary caregiver, do not forget to look after yourself as well as the primary caregiver...even if they do not ask for it or think they do not need it.

At some point in this journey, the fear I felt about all my mom was going through began to mirror my fear for dad's health. He was sleep deprived because mom woke him up throughout the nights with a flashlight in his face and strange hallucinations. He was unsettled because he never knew from minute to minute if mom would consider him a friendly face or the enemy. He was weary of if she would become combative if she did not know him. He was emotionally exhausted from watching his wife of 50 years battle a demon he could not see or protect against. He was physically exhausted because he was dedicating his days and nights to caring for his wife rather than himself.

My dad is generally an upbeat and happy guy, so when his high spirits start to wane, it is cause for concern. As a daughter, it was important for me to be there for him to be a safe place for him to vent. There were many days when he would leave mom with a professional caregiver and simply drive down the street to the neighborhood park where he would sit in his car just talking to me over the phone letting out the tears, emotions and heartache building up inside him. He no longer had his wife and built-in best friend to share his burdens with, so I did my best to step up. While he was still heartbroken and bone weary at the end of our calls, there was also a pronounced sense of relief that left him ready to return home, pick up the mantle and carry on.

In learning more about this disease and people who care for those affected by LBD, it seems as though family and friends are sorted into two primary camps. First, there are those who are willing to come alongside patients and caregivers to help them deal with the good, the bad and the ugly no matter how scared they are or what it costs them. The second group is comprised of individuals who love the patient and caregiver desperately but will isolate themselves as much as possible from the heartache of it all because they are completely overwhelmed.

I fall into the first camp. There has never been a day throughout my mom's journey with LBD that I have not been literally scared to death. I have had sleepless nights, experienced heart pounding nightmares, felt too miserable to eat, eaten too much because I'm miserable and experienced debilitating anxiety. (In full disclosure, I sometimes still do.) But never once did I consider closing up shop because it got too real.

As I've participated in support groups and spoken with other caregivers, I realize that not everyone would do what I did. It has taken a lot of time and soul searching for me to realize that my chosen way is not the only way to deal with the situation. While I may not understand how some people can turn away from instead of run toward a breaking heart, I do understand that most of those individuals can love a person just as completely and devotedly. Just differently.

I do encourage you to be involved in some way, however that looks for you. If being the caregiver who regularly interacts with the loved one is not something you feel equipped to do, then volunteer to help manage things like doctor appointments, home care and meals at a distance. Or consider showing your appreciation to the active caregiver by sending them care packages or gift cards for a dinner out. Even if you do not wish to be there in person, you can still be present in other ways.

For me, at the end of my mom's journey, I think I will be able to look back with mostly no regrets because I spent as much time with her as I possibly could, even though much of that time the woman I was with did not know me or act like my mom. I still believe that somewhere deep inside the woman my mom has become, she can still experience peace and love from regular visits and hearing I love you's. Believing that she is able to gain some sort of comfort from that makes every visit all the more worth it in my eyes.

Chapter 5

Your Name Is Not Important

I remember vividly the first time I was at my parents' house talking to my mom and she asked who I was. I would be lying if I said my heart didn't break in two that day. After all, the last time I saw her, she knew my name and that I was her daughter of more than 40 years. How do you forget something like that? The answer, of course, is that she did not forget. Lewy body dementia (LBD) took it from her.

Sometimes it would take just a small reminder to mom of who I was to her and my name, and she would fall into a comfortable conversation and enjoy our time together (although I don't think she really knew me as much as she recognized me as someone safe). Other times, I would provide her with the same information, and she would eye me as though I might be trying to pull a fast one.

My first thought was to put together a small picture album. I bought a little four by six-inch photo album at our local drug store and put a picture of each family member inside. Then I took a label maker a friend had bought me years earlier and made labels with each person's name that I affixed to each picture. Given her tendency to misplace and lose things since the dementia symptoms started in earnest, I eventually made her several of these albums, just in case. I was convinced I had solved that particular problem and thought myself wise to have made extra albums. Pride really does come before the fall because that accomplished feeling did not last long. In a matter of two weeks, my mom lost all the albums and was not even aware she had done so.

In much the same vein, we brought out old family albums that my mom spent months scrapbooking just years earlier. Surely

DOI: 10.4324/9781003656890-7

seeing her own handwriting and herself in the pictures would help her remember and bring forth feelings of joy and safety. Sadly, it did neither of those things. Instead, it only provoked her into thinking we were trying to trick her into thinking that we were her family.

I hit two brick walls in just under a month. I did not know where to go from there.

My efforts were never so made in hopes my mom would remember me one last time. I made peace with that after the first time she forgot my name. She literally could not help it, and I needed to get over it. Even though the photo albums did not work, they were intended to be a way for her to find peace and know that even if she knew nothing else, the people around her now loved her dearly.

About 95% of the time, my mom did not know my name or that I was her daughter. However, in the beginning and on the good days, she would often think I was a close friend, a sister (which she does not have) or even a kind stranger. I learned to treasure those moments because if I couldn't be her daughter, I would take any of those other scenarios in a heartbeat if it meant she would trust me and feel safe in my company. Each of those moments was a gift.

Having been through this firsthand, I do realize how traumatic it can be to have a loved one forget your name. It is gut wrenching to say the least – like someone ripped the rug right out from underneath you. But...I realized that for myself I had two options. One, I could continually cry because she did not know my name and in the process make something she could not help infinitely harder on her and I. Or, two, I could accept that our relationship went deeper than just a name and that I could bring her comfort by simply being whoever she thought I was that day if it brought her happiness amidst this awful disease.

I readily admit that I experienced that first option for maybe a week after it happened. Then I decided it was not doing her, or I, any favors and it was time to move past it. So, I did. Please note that I do not claim to have done it gracefully, but I persevered so she and I could still enjoy spending time together. So can you.

There are scores and scores of books written about what neurologists and psychologists believe happens inside a person's brain when they have a memory disease. I have read quite a few of them myself and have even have some on my nightstand now. Some of these reads are clinically based and others explore what may be happening in the brains of patients with advanced memory disease that science cannot yet explain.

Though I am not a doctor, I believe the tone and timbre of our voices still resonate with our loved ones. There have been little one to five second pockets of time throughout my mom's diagnosis where she has briefly remembered, and I believe that is because I never stopped talking to her and spending time with her. I believe our voices and actions carry far greater weight with our loved ones than they may have the capacity to acknowledge.

This is why we must continue to show up for our loved ones every day. Whether they know our names or not, I believe somewhere deep inside they still recognize our love and benefit from receiving it.

Chapter 6

Music Can Be Healing

Have you noticed how listening to just the right song can impact your mood and thoughts? Maybe you have a song you like to listen to on road trips with the sunroof open and the wind whipping through your hair. Maybe you have a go-to tune that you like to listen to when you are feeling sad. Maybe you have music you listen to when you are studying. Many of us have songs that essentially come together to form the soundtrack of our lives.

While the song you listen to on a road trip may be the perfect music for the occasion, there is a good chance you associate that song with a positive memory that further contributes to making it your song of choice in that moment.

I firmly believe that music can do wonders for memory recall... at almost any age.

For several years, I taught preschool and transitional kindergarten at a church. Part of the weekly curriculum was chapel time during which the children sang songs with Mr. Gary. While Mr. Gary did not have a fancy record label, he was most definitely a rock star to the kids and teachers he did chapel with every week. He had a beautifully unique way of pairing Scripture with upbeat music and interesting narratives to help kids remember Bible verses and be able to recall them when needed. I have not taught at that school in more than six years and Mr. Gary has since passed, but I remember many of the verses and songs we sang together and still sing them to myself today.

On the other end of the age spectrum, I remember being at a sing-along in my mom's memory care home. I couldn't help thinking it was almost cruel to ask people who could not remember how to get dressed by themselves to sing songs when the opening

DOI: 10.4324/9781003656890-8

bars of "This Little Light of Mine" filled the room. To my aston-ishment, a group of almost 20 residents of the memory care home started humming together in perfect unison. Even more amazing to me was that some of the patients were actually able to recall and sing the words. I was rendered completely speechless at how so many who hardly even spoke were able to recall the tune to this popular childhood song. Perhaps even more impressive were the smiles it brought to their faces.

With these two real-life scenarios in mind, I absolutely believe that the right music can be healing for the human spirit.

As a young girl, I remember spending many car rides listen-ing to some of my mom's favorite artists like Elvis Presley, Neil Sedaka and The Beach Boys. Because I associate these songs with happy times and often heard them on repeat, I still remember most of their words today. Their music made her happy, and I now associate these musicians and their songs with her, which makes me happy when I hear them. To this day, when I go visit my mom at memory care, I like to crank up some sixties music which features many of these artists, hoping it brings her a smile even if it is one I can't see.

In the beginning of my mom's journey with Lewy body demen-tia (LBD), she struggled with high blood pressure and anxiety that can come along with the disease. Some days she had so much pent-up energy from anxiety that it felt like she was vibrating from the inside out and virtually nothing seemed to calm her. We were not sure what to do to help.

As luck would have it, my dad connected with Mr. Gary through a Bible study, and when he explained the situation, Mr. Gary suggested incorporating music into her routine for a calming effect. Dad put together a playlist for my mom on Alexa with all her favorites across different genres. He showed her how to start her playlist so she could listen to it whenever she wanted. It worked beautifully. Certain songs seemed to level out her blood pressure while visibly taking her mind off of her anxiety. Before long, she started associating certain songs on the playlist with specific parts of her routine. It helped form and shape her day.

I remember one day in particular when I arrived for a visit, and she was dancing in the kitchen to music. I had barely cleared the door when she grabbed my hand for an impromptu dance party.

Her smile and energy were contagious. I would have bottled it if I could. That was a great day!

One way of incorporating music into your loved one's routine can be to play a series of songs for wake-up, meals, certain activities and bedtime. After a week or more of this exposure, you may find that your voice cues for certain activities are no longer needed to the extent that they were before. This can ease feelings of tension that sometimes develop between a caregiver and the patient as well as evoke feelings of peace.

If you have not yet incorporated music into your loved one's routine, it might be worth a try. It may be best to use musical favorites from their younger years or whatever time period they believe they are currently in. If your cable or streaming service has music channels, put one on from a decade your loved one remembers fondly and have it play in the background.

Do not underestimate what music can do for you as a caregiver. When you have some downtime, put in some earbuds and listen to music that brings you joy. For much of my mom's journey, I had just about anything from For King & Country on repeat because their music lifted me up at a time when I desperately needed it. They are still a favorite of mine today.

Be intentional with bringing music into the life of your loved one as well as your own and let it bring you peace and comfort that can be hard to find in dealing with LBD.

Chapter 7

Expect Visual Changes

I never anticipated the visual disturbances Lewy body dementia (LBD) would bring. Sheer ignorance and unfamiliarity with the disease had me focused on memory and cognitive issues only. I do not remember any of the educational literature I initially read talking about visual issues, but it was definitely something my mom experienced and still does to this day.

Perhaps the most notable visual changes she encountered early on was seeing multiple of one person and believing each had a different personality. For mom, it started with the person she was most familiar with, my dad, her husband of 50 years.

There were days when they would be in the same room having a conversation about a trip they had once taken together, and, almost on a dime, my mom would ask him how he knew about such things since she went with her husband and not him. Misidentification of familiar people is common in LBD because this illness causes deterioration in the parts of the brain that allow us to recognize others (see Part 1). For the majority of the time since the severe memory symptoms started, mom remained in flux about who my dad really was. Everything from leaving and reentering a room to taking a car ride and then coming back home could be a trigger for confusion. We eventually learned that occasionally the same situations that triggered her confusion could also be used to help her recognize dad again.

Just as she frequently saw multiple of my dad, we noticed it also translated to physical objects. For example, if she was making a grocery list and had a pad of paper and a pen laying on the kitchen table, when she grabbed for the pen, her hand would go to a space adjacent to the actual object. At first, I wondered if it

DOI: 10.4324/9781003656890-9

could simply be a depth perception issue, but when she asked why we had so many pens on the table and I saw only one, I realized her brain must be creating multiple images of one pen.

She frequently told us she was experiencing floating black spots in her line of vision. Early on, she attributed them to the beginnings of a migraine, but the migraine never came. It escalated when she began to complain that when she watched television, black spots distorted the picture. No one else could see them but her. One afternoon when we were watching a television show together, she questioned why the television had suddenly gone black and white when it used to show color. Just as before, she was the only one to see this phenomenon.

After a while, my mom stopped mentioning the black spots. Instead, a new visual change developed. She was seeing spots of yellow in her beige bathroom sink. According to her, the spots simply would not go away, even with strong cleaning solutions. Mom complained so often that my dad finally acquiesced to having someone come out and check the water. Unfortunately, the company that came used the opportunity to tell my parents all the things that were "wrong" with their water instead of admitting they did not see the yellow spots mom spoke of. Not cool.

Eventually, mom quit mentioning the yellow spots in the bathroom sink and instead began seeing patches of that same color on her light blue bedspread and the brown carpet. Dad and I could not see any of the yellow spots she pointed out, but "cleaned" the carpet and rewashed the bedspread in an effort to mollify her. It worked for a short time, but then she began seeing the same spots again. It is hard to talk to patients with LBD out of their false beliefs or visual disturbances. Our response was to distract and redirect when possible, rather than contradict her.

After experiencing so many issues with what we thought was my mom's vision, dad decided to take her to the ophthalmologist. While the doctor did not see anything that would cause color variations or multiple images of people or things, he did note she was developing cataracts and suggested doing the surgery might help (she wore contacts although she recently switched to glasses). Mom grew frustrated that he could not find what was causing her vision issues and the doctor was somehow increasingly unavailable when she wanted to make another appointment. Also not cool.

In the end, my parents elected to move forward with cataract surgery in both eyes through a different provider and do one eye at a time with two weeks of recuperation in between. Once both eyes had been operated on, she no longer needed to wear contacts. She still required reading glasses, yet she tended to wear them all the time.

Our hope was that the cataract surgery would correct her vision, and while it likely did, it did not correct the floating black spots, splashes of yellow or multiple images. In this respect, she remained frustrated. This correction never happened because all of these false images were generated in the brain, not the eye.

Visual hallucinations are also extremely common with this illness. Hallucinations are often lumped in with other visual disturbances in LBD. However, hallucinations are technically not so much an issue with vision as they are issues with projections of the brain. Mom's hallucinations ranged from seeing strange people in her home to seeing people sitting in parked cars outside to emergency personnel working an accident.

In the beginning, dad and I did not handle the hallucinations well. Frankly, we did not yet know any better. We were intent on showing mom that the strange people and scary things she saw were not real. We even went so far as to take a picture of what she was seeing so she could confirm it did not appear in the picture she took. Neither of these efforts worked.

As the disease progressed and we were able to find more resources on all that can come with LBD, we realized it would be better to simply distract or redirect mom when she had a hallucination. One late afternoon, my kids were with my parents at a park watching a deer grazing in the grass. My mom saw a woman feeding the deer that no one else did. When she asked my daughter if she saw it, my daughter simply said yes and then my dad changed the subject. It was enough to mollify my mom, and their afternoon continued on without an emotional blowup from a debate about whether a woman was really feeding the deer or not.

I found visual disturbances to be a hard part of this disease because although I have no doubt my mom really did see what she was telling us, we could not see it. I cannot imagine how fearful and unsure that made her feel when we verbalized that to her.

The purpose of this chapter is not necessarily to tell you that your loved one will experience visual disturbances. I am not a doctor or medical professional and cannot speak to whether everyone with LBD experiences the same phenomena. Instead, I am sharing this with you so that in the event that your loved one does encounter visual changes amidst this disease, you will know you are not alone in this.

Chapter 8

Embrace Love and Ditch Logic

I am somewhere in between a Type A and Type B personality. I do love me some organization and control, and I can do some mad research, but my mom's diagnosis taught me there are times where those qualities don't necessarily serve a dementia caregiver well.

Personally, I do much better knowing what I am up against than entering into it blindly, probably because it gives me a false sense of control. Sometimes I have a bad habit of assuming others feel the same way, when in fact they do not. Or in this case, maybe they cannot.

My mom began displaying symptoms of Lewy body dementia (LBD) well before we were able to get an official diagnosis. Unfortunately, we didn't know anything about this disease or its symptoms. So, to my family, it was almost as if mom involuntarily abandoned her life and logic overnight. Amidst all of this, the challenge became to embrace love and ditch logic. This was particularly difficult for me because ditching logic counters my natural tendencies. It took me a while to learn and accept this way of thinking when it came to caregiving.

For example, months before the official diagnosis came, my mom asked me if we could get out for a short while. This usually meant taking a drive as she did not like going inside places much anymore. So, I took her to the Chick-fil-A drive-thru for a soda and chocolate chip cookie (her favorites) before going to sit in an empty church parking lot close to my parents' home to just visit.

What I thought would be a nice mother-daughter chat quickly went downhill. That morning my dad had gotten out some cherished photo albums to show her pictures of their lives together

DOI: 10.4324/9781003656890-10

over the past five decades from dating to grandchildren. She did not remember me or my dad.

What was intended to logically show mom she could trust the pictures backfired royally. One of the primary symptoms of this type of dementia is coming up with entertaining conspiracy theories (these are called false beliefs or delusions by medical practitioners). This was on full display in that moment. Rather than logically assuming that the pictures were of her life and we were who we said we were, she wanted to know why we went to such lengths to make a photo album just to trick her into believing she was married and had children.

I remember being speechless, something that is rare for me. Of all the things she could have told me that day, I did not see this line of thought coming. It totally blindsided me. I honestly was not even sure what to reply with. Probably for that reason, I went with trying to explain to her we would never do such a thing, and that the album really was a collection of pictures from her life. I went with logic. I chose wrong. The more I worked to convince her that what I said was true, the more agitated and upset she became.

Looking back, if I really put myself in her shoes, I think I can almost imagine how this must have felt for my mom. Her brain literally wiped out the memories she had beyond her teenage years, in turn making her feel like she was still a teenager. Therefore, the memories we showed her could not possibly have happened. I would be completely frustrated if I believed the same and someone tried to tell me different. At some point, I would probably even begin to question my safety with those same people.

What I should have done was meet her where she was in that moment with love. She really was not looking for answers or logic. She was seeking love and safety. And I failed her. I thought logic would help, but it only made it worse. Speaking logic was my way of helping her when all she wanted was comfort.

Although there are new resources on different types of dementia every day, most of the information you will find about using love over logic comes from other caregivers who have walked in your shoes. "If you know, you know," as they say.

Another time when logic failed me, I explained to mom she was already at home when she did not recognize it. I explained how she had lived there 30 years and that the clothes in the closet really were hers, but to no avail. She became convinced someone was trying to duplicate her real house to trick her. Every time she asked me to take her home, I would try to explain she was already there.

Eventually I learned that, for my mom, a more prudent option than logic was to tell her that there was too much traffic on the road to leave at that time or that we would leave in the morning because it was too late to travel. Most of the time, both of these responses worked and in a way that did not make it seem as though I was disbelieving or unintentionally belittling her. The answer calmed her and in just a few hours she forgot about it entirely, or at least until we repeated the whole process again because she forgot that she ever even asked.

Many times, the alternate reality that dementia creates for a person does not have a place for logic, but it does have a place for love. Making sure your person knows they are being cared for and loved is far more important than being right, even if that comes from a place of love too.

Chapter 9

Be Proactive Because Things Will Go Missing

For most types of memory diseases, it is not a matter of if things will go missing but when. Much of the time this is because a person misplaces them, hides them or puts them in the trash. Keep in mind, these acts are seldom committed in plain view of others but rather in a furtive, private way. This means caregivers may not learn about them until sometime later when recovery of said items becomes either irrelevant or near impossible.

There is a fine line that must not be crossed when being proactive to keep things from going missing. It requires a balance between respecting a person's dignity while also protecting things you know your loved one would ultimately hate to lose if their memory was not impaired. As caregivers, you will have to tread carefully and considerately.

In light of this, it may not prove helpful to struggle with items that can be easily replaced. For example, a new universal remote can usually be purchased if one is lost. If pens, pencils and notepads that your loved one uses to make notes seem to keep walking away, they can easily be repurchased. Items such as these are generally not worth worrying about losing in the grand scheme of things.

However, items such as important papers, smartphones, driver's licenses, wallets and jewelry are more critical and cannot be as easily replaced. These should be proactively safeguarded as once they go missing, the reality is that you may not ever get them back.

One of the most prominent conspiracy theories of people with memory disease is that people are stealing from them. As incorrect as they may be, the patient generally feels as though it is

DOI: 10.4324/9781003656890-11

very real. For that reason, they will take steps to safeguard their important things. Unfortunately, this can result in them hiding objects in potentially unsafe places. One staff person at a memory home I toured told me it was not uncommon for dementia patients to flush some items down the toilet thinking the objects would be safer there.

In reality, caregivers will be unable to keep some items from becoming lost. This would require making caregiving a full-time job in which you are never out of sight to go to the restroom, another room or even focus on the television. Even if you could manage somehow to be present around the clock without breaks, your presence would likely increase agitation in your loved one therefore making it almost counterproductive.

The alternative is to be proactive. While there are no one-size-fits-all methods for doing this, here are a few helpful ideas that others have shared with me and that I have found helpful along the way.

Important Papers

These can include bills, doctor's notes, MRI orders and wills. If any of these items go missing, it has the potential to thoroughly derail a person's life. The best way to protect these papers may be to put them in a fire and waterproof safe that can only be accessed by key. This type of safe is generally heavy enough to keep a person from picking it up and toting it around. It is big enough that it cannot be easily hidden. Finally, it cannot be opened without a key which your loved one should not have access to.

If the person becomes agitated and securing these items becomes a catalyst for confrontation, then consider leaving blank or "dummy" papers in the places where these important papers would normally be stored. This can give your loved one a sense of agency and independence as they are still able to shuffle papers to their heart's content without risking the safety of the real documents.

Smartphones and Cell Phones

For many patients with dementia, smartphones or cell phones can become a source of paranoia. This usually takes the form of fixating on others' phones rather than their own simply because many forget how to use them. In terms of your loved one's phone, it may be helpful to replace a smartphone with a more limited functioning phone to reduce accidental purchases and phone calls. Low-end phones designed for limited capabilities are not as expensive to replace as regular smartphones and cell phones.

In terms of your own smartphone, I strongly suggest keeping it on your person at all times or it may end up missing. My mom was often bothered if my dad was on the phone. She dreamed up conspiracy theories constantly about who he was texting or talking to when he was usually just playing games or speaking with me. For this reason, if he left his phone sitting on a table or desk, he could count on it to go missing because she hid it somewhere. The moral of the story is not to leave your phone unattended.

Driver's Licenses and Wallets

Someone once told me her husband simply could not bear to be without the cards in his wallet because it was a form of independence for him. She found this out when she removed the cards from his wallet to keep him from losing them and he melted down. Her solution was to make a paper copy of his driver's license (he was no longer driving) and put it in his wallet along with some old gift cards.

This seemed like an ingenious idea to me because it kept the patient from losing important items. If a credit card were to be lost and you did not know about it, you would not know to cancel it. Should the card fall into the wrong hands, this could result in thousands of dollars of credit card debt. Even though a person is no longer driving, if their driver's license is lost, they would be without ID for medical procedures and such.

Let your loved one carry a wallet that is inexpensive and fill it with old gift cards and maybe a few one-dollar bills so they still feel as though they have a real wallet even though the things in it are largely not functional.

Jewelry

This is a big one, especially for the ladies. I'll be honest, my family waited too long on this front and as a result some of my mom's nicest pieces of jewelry have become forever lost. And when I say lost, I mean gone. I went through my parents' house with a fine-tooth comb checking between and under furniture cushions, boxes in the pantry, the back of drawers, rolled up socks, clothes pockets and so on. I did find quite a few things that had been hidden in weird places, but none of her missing jewelry.

I am not even sure how expensive the jewelry was. I only know that it was important to her, which makes it important to me.

Do not wait too late. If there is a special family heirloom, store it in a safety deposit box or somewhere safe because if you don't, your loved one may unintentionally dispose of it or hide it somewhere it cannot be found.

Be as proactive as you can in protecting your loved one's most treasured possessions while also keeping their dignity intact, for your sake and theirs.

Chapter 10

Home Is Where the Heart Is

Whether it is Lewy body dementia (LBD), Alzheimer's or another memory disease, it is common to hear a caregiver talk about how their loved one who currently resides at home keeps asking to be taken home. What I came to learn is that home is where the heart is, and for a person with dementia, that is often in a time period other than the current one.

In the very beginning, my mom thought she was living in an apartment and going between it and her home. In reality, she was still living in her home of 30 plus years and never left. Nevertheless, she was certain she was traveling between two places of residence. A few months later, the conspiracy theories that frequently come with LBD began to take over. Mom thought the place she was living had been created to look like her "real" home. There was no point in arguing because she firmly believed we were part of a plan designed to deceive her. This type of false belief is called reduplicative paramnesia by specialists and is common in LBD.

As a result of this revolving concept of home, mom was constantly packing, unpacking or repacking a tote bag, duffel bag or purse (or all three). It is worth noting here that my mom has always loved purses and bags, so in a way this was likely a natural comfort zone for her. Still, it created problems. She had close to a dozen purses and tote bags combined, and when she was constantly transferring her belongings from one to the other, the end result was at least six partially packed bags with a couple of items in each. When you consider that she did this multiple times a day every day, it should come as no surprise that she started misplacing and losing her belongings. This created an extra level of chaos.

DOI: 10.4324/9781003656890-12

There were times when mom would be content watching television or having a conversation, only to suddenly straighten up and say she wanted to go home right away before she left the room to pack her bags. This usually occurred without a natural trigger. It just happened and we were clueless as to why.

Before we knew better, we tried to convince mom she was at home and explain our reasoning. Unfortunately, logic was not helpful in this situation. It only managed to make her more fearful and convinced her we were all in league to keep her from her real home.

One day I asked mom if she could tell me where home was. She did not hesitate to share that home was in a different city where she grew up with her parents and brother. Didn't I remember the street name? Weren't her parents worried about her? How long would it take to get there?

My mom's parents passed a decade or more before her diagnosis. Her childhood home was sold before her dad ever passed. There was no childhood home to go back to. We realized none of these conversations would be helpful to have with her, nor would she be able to understand them. With a little help from other caregivers, we learned to tell her it was too late to travel and that we would go first thing in the morning, by which time she would have forgotten the conversation had ever taken place. Other times, we would tell her that it was rush hour and traffic was too heavy to travel right then. This explanation worked much the same way.

Of all the issues not being able to recognize home can cause for a person with memory issues, two of the more serious problems are not accessing the amenities and attempting to escape. Both can be quite serious and should be anticipated before they become a problem.

For my mom, not accessing the amenities of home affected her daily needs being met. There were times when she would not retrieve food from the pantry or refrigerator because she thought she did not live there and did not want to be accused of stealing food. The result was that she would skip meals unless someone she trusted as a "friendly" person (because she did not know us) presented her with a meal "sent" by the people who owned the place where she was staying.

Some days she would claim the washer and dryer were "different" than the one at her home and that she did not know how to use them. The simple solution would have been to let my dad do the laundry for her, but she was seldom open to that arrangement since it would take away the independence of doing that chore on her own. Many times, the solution that worked the best was myself or a respite caregiver going on an outdoor walk with her while my dad started a load of laundry. By the time mom got back to the house, she had forgotten about the washer entirely.

When a person with a memory disease believes they are being made to stay somewhere that is not home, they may attempt to escape. It could even make some individuals feel like they have been kidnapped.

There are several different approaches to this scenario and every family should choose what they believe is in the best interest of their loved one. For example, some families may simply alert their neighbors to the situation and ask them to be secondary lookouts for their loved one. Others may choose to put deadbolts on exterior doors so that a key is required, and the individual cannot walk out of the house at night while their caretaker is sleeping unaware.

While each family must decide what they believe to be the right path forward, there is one piece of wisdom I will offer. One day we had an issue where my mom walked out the back door after returning from an outing and went to a neighbor's house to call the authorities because she did not recognize her home or her husband. Both the EMT and police officers who came told us they could only respond to incidents like these so many times before firmly recommending relocating the affected individual to a care facility.

These were certainly not easy words to hear, but I am thankful they were shared. This spurred us to seek professional caregiving help at home, a medical identification bracelet for my mom and more as a safety net. Then, when we knew the time had finally come, we transferred mom to a memory care facility because we believed it was truly in her best interest.

My best advice is to remember that home is where the heart is. If your loved one thinks home is somewhere else other than where they live, invite them to tell you about it and why it makes them happy. Meet them where they are as best you can.

Chapter 11

Changes May Be Needed

There were times when my dad and I were so overwhelmed with all the things that came with a Lewy body dementia (LBD) diagnosis, we found it difficult to recognize when other changes needed to be made in order to help my mom.

Driving was a big change. While mom had not driven anywhere since the diagnosis, it became clear that in the moments she failed to recognize the person she was with at home, she might be tempted to try to flee in her car. Granted, at this stage in her diagnosis, it became unlikely that she would know how to even start the car. Still, it was a risk we were not willing to take. The answer was obvious. It was time to take away the car keys.

Since I am the daughter and secondary caregiver, much of this burden fell directly on my dad's shoulders. He simply told mom that he and the doctor determined it was not safe for her to drive anymore. It is an understatement to say it infuriated her. She was resentful toward my father (and me, because in her mind I was guilty by association) and would tell anyone willing to listen that we were crazy because she was just fine to be driving. I am not sure she ever quite got over having the privilege of driving taken away from her, but as it was for her own safety and those of others, it had to be done.

It is one thing to have the privilege to drive and not use it and then quite another to not have the option. This was a huge hit to her self-sufficiency, and I really felt for her, although not enough to reverse dad's and my decision. Looking back, I'm sure she saw it as just another way the disease eroded her joy and independence.

DOI: 10.4324/9781003656890-13

In the years before my mom displayed symptoms of dementia, one of her favorite things to do on a cool fall afternoon was to take a good book and sit at our local Sonic with the windows down sipping on a Vanilla Diet Coke. She treasured that quiet time and enjoyed the cooler weather while reading a sweet romance novel. I know beyond a shadow of a doubt that when her keys were taken away, this was the activity she grieved the most. I took her on several occasions to do this same activity, but it was not quite the same for her.

While it was difficult to endure her frustration and see her heartache, there was never a question that in her specific situation, taking away the keys to the car was the right thing to do. Sometimes doing what is right is not fun but necessary – for the person suffering from dementia as well as others.

As LBD gained a greater foothold, we noticed my mom constantly losing or misplacing things. However, in her mind, most of the time she was just putting items in a safe place. There were whole days spent turning the house upside down looking for a remote, the phone or her wallet which we would find only to repeat it again the next day. It wore all of us down.

My husband did some research and came up with the idea of using Tiles. This line of products is designed to help a person locate something that has been lost, stolen or misplaced. They come in the form of stickers, cards for the wallet, keyrings and more. You can then connect these things to a caregiver's smartphone so that they are able to track the items when lost. It made finding lost items a little easier and in half the time. Now, there are many providers of services like this one, so choose one that works for your family.

Groceries were another area that required change. For as long as I can remember, mom kept a notepad on the side of the refrigerator where she would write down items needed on the next grocery run. With COVID-19 and her LBD diagnosis, my parents still made their list the same way but opted to do curbside pickup. This allowed them to drive over and pick up the groceries and then go home to unload them together. The day my dad found a package of ground meat in mom's closet, he knew he needed to start unloading the groceries solo. Again, I do not believe, in this instance, that she was trying to hide food or be sneaky.

I think she put the meat where her brain told her it needed to go. From that point on, it became common practice to distract mom when dad came home with groceries so he could unload items and make sure they made it to their rightful places, at least for the time being.

Cooking became another area that necessitated change. Although mom never really loved to cook, it became even more pronounced with the onset of LBD. Mom seldom made a meal anymore (and never alone) for fear she would leave the oven or stove on. However, even the cognitive work it took to gather the ingredients for a meal and cook it was just too much. As a result, dad did his best to have fully cooked food accessible to her in the refrigerator.

Yet, there came a time when even that method presented challenges. Laying a cooked hotdog on a bun and putting it in the microwave for a minute and then trying to add mustard and shredded cheese was a huge undertaking for her that would take half an hour. While it would have been easier for dad or I to just make the meal for her, being present and overseeing her put it together gave her an important sense of independence that was worth the 30 minutes. It was a change we were happy to make to bring her some much-needed satisfaction.

Laundry had never been a favorite chore of my mother's, but it became such after her diagnosis. It was almost an addiction for her as she would do multiple loads a day, sometimes with only a couple of items in each. The problem came not with using the right settings for the washer and dryer but with her trusting the timer. A load would be in the washer for five minutes, and even though the timer said there was 45 minutes of wash time left, my mom thought the timer and washer were broken because the clothes were still soggy and soapy. The timer was also an issue with the dryer. She felt certain that the dryer was broken because after the five minutes that she thought were an hour, the clothes were still not dry.

Because doing laundry had become a source of purpose for her, my dad and I tried to hang around when she was setting the machines and then keep her busy while they were doing what washers and dryers do. Then when the clothes and towels were dry, we enlisted her help in folding and hanging up the clothes as it still gave her a feeling of autonomy over the process.

Hands down, one of the biggest trials for my dad was keeping up with paperwork needed for bill paying, receipts, medical forms and so on because mom would constantly relocate them or throw them away thinking they were trash. There were countless times he thought he'd found the perfect place to store important papers where she would never find them, but she did. He found the answer to be purchasing a small document safe for which he kept the key. This turned out to be a godsend because we didn't have to go on a scavenger hunt looking for important papers she needed for an MRI or other procedure when it was time for an appointment.

The bottom line is that LBD (and most memory disease diagnoses) will require changes. Expect this going forward so it is not a surprise. Acknowledge this is the path before you as a caregiver and then come up with best possible resolution for you and your loved one.

I do not like change. It is a weakness for me, so I understand why mom did not love it either. But I had peace when I laid my head on my pillow each night knowing changes were made for mom's good, even if she hated us for it. Doing the right thing is not always easy but necessary.

Chapter 12

The Effects of Changing Your Loved One's Location

Once I thought I had a grasp on the fact that my mom no longer remembered who my dad and I were and that she did not always remember where she was, a new challenge came into the picture. It seemed that by simply changing my mom's location, even from room to room, it had the potential to make her forget who and what was in the previous room.

It is almost as difficult to explain as it is to understand, so I will rely on examples to illustrate what I mean.

A simple car ride had the power to alter my mom's state of mind. For example, if she got in the car with me and we went to lunch, when it was time to leave and get back in the car to go home, she suddenly did not know me. Sometimes she would be straightforward in telling me she did not recognize me. Other days she would simply stare quizzically at my face like she could not quite place me. Nothing had changed other than our location, but it was enough to create significant ripple effects.

My mom could be in a room with my dad watching television and then become wildly confused after awaking from a nap on the couch. When she went to bed, my dad was my dad or at least someone she recognized as a nice person. After she woke up, she was often angry and fearful at his presence and did not recognize him as familiar or friendly. Again, the only thing that changed was her location.

Even a car ride to the grocery store to pick up curbside could quickly go awry. When my mom and dad left the house to pick up groceries, all seemed fine. By the time they parked at the curbside area less than ten minutes away, mom no longer knew who he was. She got out of the car and adamantly refused to get back

DOI: 10.4324/9781003656890-14

in. At this point, the only thing left for him to do was call me to meet them to see if she recognized me and would get in my car. Fortunately, it did work the time or two we were forced to resort to this.

My parents still lived in the two-story house I grew up in. Now that my sister and I moved out and started our own families, the upstairs floor was seldom frequented. One night my mom wandered upstairs because she was convinced there were people living up there (there were not). She called me on the phone from one of the bedrooms whispering and asking where my dad was because there was a strange man downstairs that she did not know. My dad was there when she left to go upstairs, and she knew him but being separated from him even momentarily seemed to trigger a loss of memory.

For a person with Lewy body dementia (LBD), any change in their environment can have a profound impact. This means a change in location, décor or even color can affect them. I read this somewhere shortly before Christmas one year and told my dad we might need to reconsider how we decorated the house for the holidays. That time of year was always one of mom's favorites and she liked to go all out. We tried keeping the decorations to a fraction of their normal volume, but mom was not having it. In the end, we decorated near full capacity. The only real change we noticed was that the lights on the Christmas tree seemed to lend themselves to her hallucinations. That, and with the Christmas lights up on the exterior of the house, she frequently "saw" people gathered outside on the street, and she would sit on the couch looking out the windows to watch.

Even taking her from the house on a car ride became an issue, thanks to an uptick in hallucinations while in the car. Driving her to a hair appointment one time, she called out in alarm thinking she saw someone running out in front of my car. It scared me as the driver. I feared for a moment that I had not seen something she did, and it panicked me. It didn't take long to realize what really happened (nothing), but I still felt shaken.

I think as caregivers, unless we realize that changing our loved one's environment or location can have a huge impact, we unintentionally set ourselves up for failure. In the beginning, I knew nothing of this until I read it on a feed somewhere which is why I'm sharing it here now with you.

Chapter 13

Holidays and Gatherings

Thanksgiving and Christmas were my mom's favorite holidays. She loved everything about them, but the best part for her was the whole family coming together under one roof. Now that I am a mom myself, I appreciate this sentiment in a whole new way.

She kicked off each holiday of the year by adding extra little touches of the season to her décor. Always organized and purposeful, the decorations went the same place year after year. For most celebrations, the décor was light but festive. The exception to the rule was Christmas. For this time of the year, she went all out.

By the time my mom received the official diagnosis of Lewy body dementia (LBD), we knew Christmas would probably look different. She frequently believed she was staying at a hotel instead of her house of 30 years therefore she was afraid to touch or move much of anything. The times she did recognize it as her own home, she felt certain things were going missing. Any lights, including regular table lamps, cast shadows that played with her vision and seemed to only breed hallucinations.

None of these new behaviors were lending themselves to her cherished tradition of decorating for Christmas. Would she want to get out the decorations? Would the lights on the Christmas tree make her hallucinations go wild and increase her anxiety? Would she end up hiding some of her decorations because she felt that would make them safer?

We decided as a family on a wait-and-see approach. If mom asked to decorate, we would suggest a more minimal approach and hope that would suffice. As it often happens with dementia, our plan did not match hers when the time came.

DOI: 10.4324/9781003656890-15

One day she asked to get the decorations down and was insistent we go full steam ahead. However, since I was in charge of unloading the decorations, I made a few modifications on the sly as we went. Not every lovey or sign came out and I pretended I could not find the stair rail greenery or lights as I felt certain they would be a problem. Of course, she found the greenery in record time, and we ended up putting it out after all.

As her daughter, I wanted to put everything up to just bring her a little bit of joy as it seemed to be currently doing, but I knew as soon as her memory and mood shifted, things had the potential to change quickly.

In the end, we traded her usual tree for a much smaller one which she, thankfully, did not seem to notice. We unpacked tree ornaments for almost a half hour before I realized that for every two ornaments I unwrapped for the tree, she unconsciously took one and wrapped it back up and returned it to the box.

The lights she was so adamant about, both inside and out, did prove to be a problem. They created shadows and inspired hallucinations, but she would not let us take them down and became agitated at just the thought. As a caregiver, you have to pick your battles, and this one was not one I wanted to fight.

Looking back, that first year was still one of her best Christmases post diagnosis. The subsequent years, she was unable to cook, understand presents or be excited as she did not recognize us as her family and did not want all the fuss she used to treasure.

For some people with memory disease, changing their regular environment in even the smallest of ways can cause them great distress. They may think someone has broken in or that the location where they are is not their home. For others, the presence of holiday decorations may be welcome at first but will become a problem later. I have found the best rule of thumb to be to meet your loved one where they are.

In addition to holiday decorations, having big groups of family and friends around can also be a trigger for anxiety, confusion and meltdowns. If the affected person lives alone or with only one other and then a group of four or more family members arrives for the day, the change in routine combined with faces that the person may or may not recognize can cause them to be highly uncomfortable.

Be prepared for this to happen. Create a quiet space in the home where your loved one can go if they are overstimulated or anxious. Try to keep noise and loud outbursts to a minimum as those will frequently startle the person. Finally, if a crowd proves to be an overwhelming trigger, consider not having so many people over at once and stagger visits over the course of a week.

There are things I wish I had known that first year, that I'm going to now pass on to you. Know that just because it did not work for my mom does not mean that it will not work for your loved one. Every person is different. Take these tips under consideration and see what works best for you and your loved one:

1 Volunteer yourself to get out the decorations. If retrieving them from a location your loved one cannot see, such as the attic, pull down just enough decorations instead of all the decorations.

2 Limit or do away with decorations that come with lights (candles, twinkle lights and so on) as they may make hallucinations worse.

3 Do not put any decorations on the floor. Even setting a figurine or stuffed animal in a place where it usually is not can become a new tripping hazard.

4 Do not move things around on the kitchen or bathroom counter as it can be quite confusing.

5 Put away boxes as soon as possible to keep the area from becoming too cluttered and your loved one becoming too frustrated.

6 Ask your loved one if they are up for company before they come over. At the very least, give them the option to retreat to their room for quiet alone time.

7 Start with small groups in advance of the big holiday celebration. This will help you gauge what to expect and make accommodations ahead of time.

8 Expect the unexpected and be ready to go with the flow.

Lastly, try to relax and enjoy the holidays yourself. If you plan ahead and accept that things will probably not go like you think they will, you are doing all you can do. Don't forget to pause and let yourself bask in the beauty of the season as you care for your loved one.

Chapter 14

A Word of Caution about Hospital Visits

Thus far, in my mom's journey with Lewy body dementia (LBD), we have had two experiences at two different hospitals. Each led me to feel that a caregiver's perspective on LBD would not be complete without addressing the subjects of ambulance transfers and hospital visits.

A fall and burgeoning bump on the head are what led to my mom's first trip to the hospital. The memory care home's protocol dictated she be taken there by ambulance. My dad and I arrived at the hospital shortly after the ambulance and found my mom in an emergency room (ER) with the lights considerably dimmed and no nurse or hospital personnel present. She was in a mobilizing neck brace.

Mom was quiet and fearful as she did not understand where she was nor could remember why she was there. After tracking down a nurse, we learned she would be in the neck brace until X-rays and scans showed it would be safe to remove it. There were no chairs in the room, so we stood by mom's bed and spoke softly which seemed to bring her some degree of comfort despite her not knowing who we were.

I will never forget a nurse coming in to give my mom a bedpan and telling her she needed a urine sample. Mom responded with a timid, "What?" The nurse repeated herself and it prompted a repeat question from my mom. This went on for ten minutes before the nurse decided to let me aid mom with it. The nurse was frustrated, as I was, but for entirely different reasons. I am not sure what she knew about dementia (much less LBD), but it was clearly not enough to realize that mom's cognitive decline did not allow her to process or follow directions well, if at all.

DOI: 10.4324/9781003656890-16

The final diagnosis was a broken collar bone and a nasty bump on the head that was thought not to be a concussion but required close monitoring. Before we ever left the hospital, we spoke to the nurse at her memory care home to ensure they would be able to sufficiently meet mom's needs as she healed. Thankfully, they were.

When we left the hospital for the memory care unit, my dad drove while I sat in the backseat with mom. This was both to keep a close eye on her and to prevent her from becoming scared and trying to open the car door while the vehicle was in motion. She had many tears and much confusion and was not open to being hugged so I spoke softly, and dad played some calming music on the radio.

Nine months later, mom fell again with a potentially fractured hip. Again, the home had the ambulance transport her to the hospital, but this time everything went downhill fairly fast.

The EMT service took mom to a different hospital than what our family and the memory care home requested, unbeknownst to all of us. After waiting for almost an hour for her to arrive at the hospital we requested, we started to wonder and began calling other hospitals to see if she had been taken somewhere else. Indeed, she had been taken to a different hospital. My dad, sister and I drove to that location to find mom was on site and in the hospital's record system. However, there were no patient rooms available, so she was forced to stay in the ambulance bay for an excruciating four hours. They were able to do much of her X-rays and scans from there, but the situation was far from ideal.

Once she made it into an ER and we could go back to be with her, I was not prepared to see what I did. Her 100-pound frame looked so tiny. Her eyes were wide with fear and her body violently shook in a way that indicated it was from far more than fear or being cold. As she shook and the nurse prepared to do an IV, I requested mom at least be given some warm blankets first so she would not be shaking as hard when they tried to put a needle in her arm.

As the nurse retrieved mom's hand from under the blanket she came into the hospital with, we (nurses included) discovered that my mom's hands had been individually bound with medical tape and far too tightly. It took two trained nurses almost ten minutes to unwrap her hands which were wrapped so compactly that her hands looked misshapen for some time. I. Was. Livid.

No wonder my poor mom was terrified. From her point of view, it probably felt akin to being bound and kidnapped given the dementia. I simply could not fathom how she must have felt.

After a somewhat heated discussion, it became clear the EMTs had wrapped her hands that way because she was trying to pull free of wires during her four-hour stay in the ambulance. While I could see how this might be a challenge for EMTs and might require some sort of action to keep a patient from hurting themselves or the equipment, if a patient's hands are wrapped so tightly that it takes two nurses ten minutes to undo, that does not even remotely indicate professionalism.

(The ongoing theme throughout this chapter is that our hospitals, doctors, nurses, EMTs and other key health professionals need access to dementia training and have it be required as part of their onboarding and professional development. An intentional ignorance of dementia, a varied condition affecting millions of adults, stands in sharp contrast to the Hippocratic Oath. Please note that I believe this starts all the way at the top in medical education and training.)

Because my dad, sister and I all stood in the room taking up space and I am sure being a bit of an inconvenience in the ER (I was glad we were), a doctor made her way over. She explained that the EMTs had to take mom to this particular hospital instead of the one we requested because it had a trauma designation and mom's fall was in that category. While I can understand and respect protocol, it should also have been protocol for the EMTs to alert the memory care home they were taking her to a different hospital and why...before they ever left the premises.

Other reasons I'm beyond grateful we were there with her included being able to request warm blankets for her chills, asking for morphine for her pain, advocating for her dementia and telling yet another nurse what I thought of him asking mom to get up and provide him a urine sample with just the look on my face. My sweet friend, Kelly, said she was sure my facial expression had captions that day!

Due to the nature of mom's health before the hip fracture and the toll anesthesia and surgeries can take on people who have LBD, our family opted to decline surgery which would require months of physical therapy (PT) for her at a facility that would likely also not understand her dementia diagnosis. We believed this type of predicament could have made a hard situation even harder on mom.

The purpose in my sharing these stories is not to scare you but to equip you for hospital stays for your loved one when they occur. Whether they are being transported from your home or a memory care unit, if their destination is a hospital, they will unequivocally need you to advocate for them in almost every way imaginable. (Please note, however, that there is a difference between responsibly advocating and being unnecessarily difficult.)

Most memory care units and nursing homes do not send a staff member to the hospital along with the patient in the ambulance. While they may clearly describe the condition of the patient to the EMTs, that service must then describe it to the hospital staff, and at some point, it can become a game of Telephone gone horribly wrong.

For this reason, if your loved one with LBD should require a hospital trip, meet them at the hospital as soon as possible. Otherwise, they will likely be alone, and with the added trauma of whatever necessitated the trip, they may be struggling even more with speaking, comprehending someone's words and any other number of cognitive abilities. They need you there to advocate for them with both nurses and doctors. Unless there is a strong understanding of LBD amongst the hospital staff, it can be best to stay with your loved one the entire time they are there. Even if one nurse is fabulous and understands exactly how to work with your loved one, there are shift changes that can take everyone back to square one.

If you are headed to the hospital, expect to be there for a while and pack accordingly. Bring your phone, a charger, snacks, books and whatever else can keep you busy while you acclimate to what I like to call hospital time. If possible, split shifts with family and friends to ease some of the burden and get a little rest.

I will say that two of the doctors throughout both hospital experiences were amazing and had an excellent handle on LBD and all the complications that can come with it. We even had a soon-to-be nurse who was simply marvellous before shift changes soon took her away.

I believe there are incredibly talented and smart people providing care in our hospitals, but I also think that those who have not seen dementia up close and personal tend to lack an adequate understanding. Sadly, this directly impacts how they care for a patient with dementia who is suffering.

Personally, I think the answer lies in properly educating and training our EMTs and medical professionals in dementia diagnoses. Organizations such as the Lewy Body Dementia Association have already started campaigns to help better educate medical professionals in this realm for which I am grateful.

There is still much work to be done in this area. If you are looking for a way to volunteer and serve, give some thought to if educating others might be a good fit for you and how you could start a program that might then be replicated on a large scale so others can implement it wherever they live. You would be changing the lives of both patients and loved ones in very significant and long-lasting ways.

Chapter 15

Love Your Person as They Are

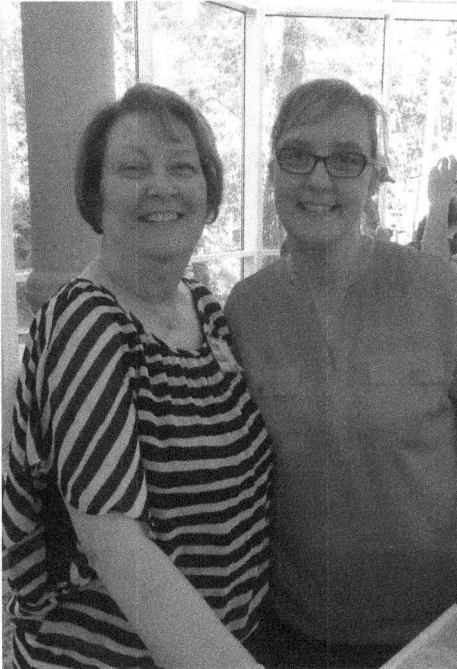

Figure 15.1 Kimberly and her mother.

DOI: 10.4324/9781003656890-17

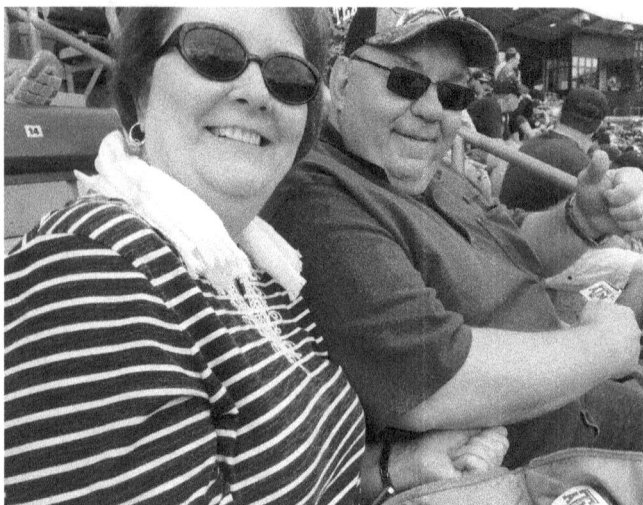

Figure 15.2 Kimberly's mother and father at a Texas A&M baseball game.

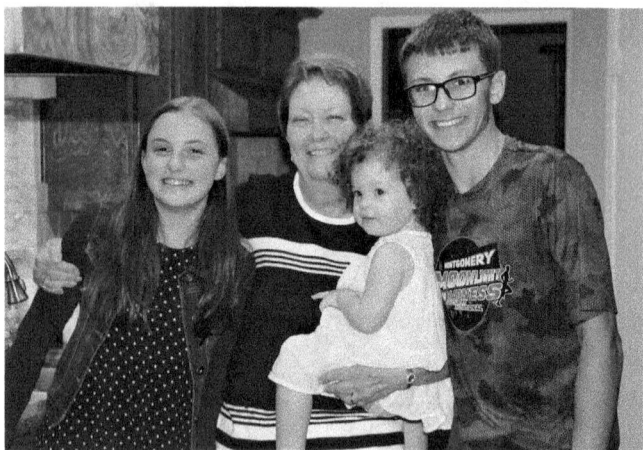

Figure 15.3 Kimberly's mother taking a break in the kitchen to pose for a picture with the grandchildren.

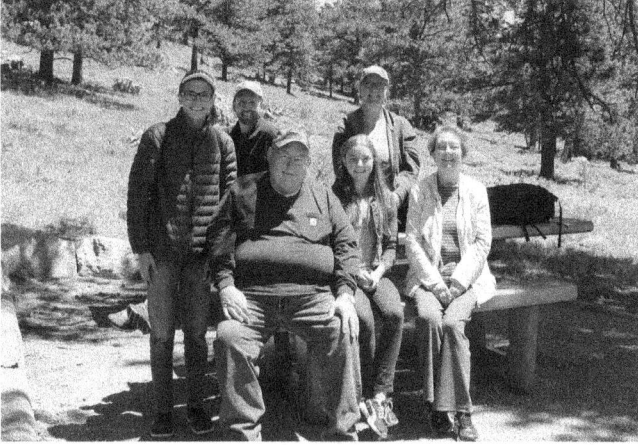

Figure 15.4 Kimberly with her son, husband, father, daughter and mother gathering around a picnic table in Rocky Mountain National Park.

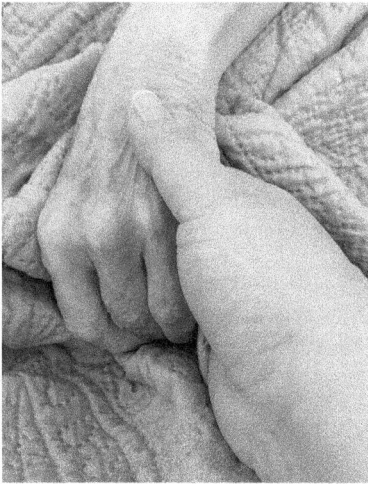

Figure 15.5 Kimberly's hand holding her mother's.

Loving your person exactly as they are is one of the most difficult rules of dementia caregiving to abide by, primarily because who they are always seems to be changing. In the beginning, it can change from week to week. As the disease progresses, it changes from day to day and sometimes hour to hour or even minute to minute. This means that loving your person as they are may require you to switch gears several times a day.

For me, the most challenging period of constant change occurred before my mom's official Lewy body dementia (LBD) diagnosis. My family had no understanding of what she was experiencing in the confines of her head or why she was experiencing it. All we could see was the outward manifestations which typically looked like vitamin deficiency, amnesia, paranoia or some combination of the three. Without proper testing or a diagnosis, it felt impossible to know how to help my mom, which only frustrated her and us (Figures 15.1–15.5).

During this season, I spent endless amounts of energy trying to convince my mom I was indeed her daughter or at least a "safe" person who loved her dearly. It was largely in vain. On the rare day that her memory did somehow manage to piece together that I was her daughter, it was gone in the matter of an hour. Without a diagnosis or any knowledge of dementia, I was bent on trying to fit her back into the box of her previous self. Now, as I look back and realize she had LBD, it breaks my heart to think how that must have made her feel. My mom did not know who she had been. So, how could she possibly become that person again?

Loving your person as they are can look different at each stage of dementia. When I look back on my mom's journey with LBD to date, this is what it looked like for us:

- Uncharacteristic Forgetfulness (pre-diagnosis). In the beginning, mom could not remember what time we had set for lunch or what date we were going to celebrate her birthday. In some ways, this stage turned out to be a blessing in disguise because it is what alerted my family to the fact that there might be a developing problem. During this stage, I remember jogging her memory about our prior conversations and thinking that would be the end of it. I was wrong. It was only the beginning. As a caregiver, I do not remember having anger but primarily bewilderment about why these changes were taking place. It is what prompted us to make an appointment with her primary doctor.

- Failed Recognition (pre-diagnosis). The instances in which my mom did not recognize my dad or I or anyone else in the family before we had an official diagnosis were the hardest because we could not understand what was happening. I think we all thought if we worked hard enough, we could just help her remember. When mom did not recognize anyone, she felt unsafe and seemed to vibrate with the anxiety of it all. None of us wanted her to feel anxious or fearful. In this stage, I do know it was less about us wanting her to remember our names or what we were to her, and more about her knowing us at least as familiar faces so she would feel safe. Loving her in this season meant not correcting her when she told us she was unmarried. It meant us not being offended when she did not know our names or roles within the family as long as she saw us as friendly, safe people.

- Pre-diagnosis Anger. There were times as the disease took hold in which my mom could become irrationally angry. I distinctly remember one evening when she called my house upset with me specifically for something that never actually happened but that her brain manufactured. My dad could not get her to take her medicine. Instead of being offended by her words and false accusations (or trying not to be anyway), I apologized and said I could understand how she would feel that way. I told her if she would take the medicine dad was trying to give her, he would also give her a pen and paper so she could make a list of the things I had done to anger her. While it was clear all was not forgotten, this seemed to satisfy her and make her feel heard. In this stage, loving mom where she was meant pushing my feelings to the side and doing what was best for her even if it meant accepting responsibility for something that never happened.

- Post-diagnosis Memory Lapses and Awareness. I think the most brutal stage for my mom was this one. I cannot fathom how horrible it must feel to have periods of knowing who you are and that you have LBD, only to realize you have had concerning episodes in which you knew neither. The memory lapses and lack of awareness also impacted her favorite activity, walking outside. She heavily resented we would not allow her to go walking by herself around the neighborhood. This was primarily because she did not remember that the previous week while walking, she started to wander off without realizing it. When we tried to explain the why of not walking by herself anymore, she cried when she realized her reality had become indistinguishable from the blank spaces in her memory. At this point, loving her where she was meant holding her as she cried and letting my own tears mingle with hers while stroking her hair.

- Post-diagnosis Hallucinations. What I would have given in this stage to know one of the worst things you can do is tell a person with LBD hallucinations that you cannot see what they see. When my mom would experience a scary hallucination, I originally thought letting her know I could not see it would calm her because she would then realize it was not real. I could not have been more wrong. It only led to her feeling as though I invalidated all she was seeing and experiencing. Now I know the key is to distract and redirect the person experiencing hallucinations. Their brain really is showing them something scary; it is not just a wild imagination. Therefore, it must be the most frustrating thing in the world for them to try to warn others of what they are seeing and have no one believe them. Eventually, I learned when mom had a hallucination, the best thing for me to do was to neither confirm nor deny the presence of something scary she saw outside. Instead, I would say something like, "Then we should probably move away from the window and go watch tv in the other room." Much of the time, this was all it took. Loving her where she was meant learning how to help, not giving her a lesson in reality.

- Post-diagnosis Favorites. Caregivers often find that they soon become persona non grata because they are viewed by the patient as a super bossy killjoy who is always hovering close by. It did not take long for my dad and I to be viewed as such by my mom. One evening my mom did not recognize my dad, even though he said he was her husband. She called me wanting confirmation that what he said was true. Although I confirmed it, she thought I was only saying what he wanted me to say. In a last ditch effort, I asked her if she wanted to ask her question to my husband for added confirmation. As soon as my husband confirmed what my dad said was true, she immediately relented and took him at his word. Loving her where she was in this stage meant connecting her with trusted family members when she wanted nothing to do with me or my dad.

- Memory Care Unit Placement. Even with the assistance of professional caregivers in my parents' house part-time, it eventually became evident my mom needed more care than what we could provide. This was a decision we did not take lightly. We wanted to keep her at home with us but ultimately realized that would be more for our own benefit than hers. Loving my mom where she was in this season meant putting her needs ahead of our wants. (All this said, I do acknowledge specialized care at a memory care unit is not affordable for everyone. To caregivers who identify with this statement, please know I see you and my heart and prayers are with you. You are amazing and your loved one is so lucky to have you.)

- Memory Care Unit Visits. Visits to the memory unit have always been a mixed bag depending on the stage my mom was in and what kind of day she was having. Now, loving her where she is at requires a great deal of flexibility and patience because much like in the very beginning, where she is mentally changes every single day. Sometimes it meant walking laps inside the home with her without talking because the exercise calmed her. Sometimes it meant playing along with wild delusions that made her happy. Other times it meant twisting my body like a pretzel just to feed her lunch (she can no longer feed herself) because she did not want to properly face me. Now, it mostly means sitting by her hospital bed at a distance because she does not like it when I draw near (her vision has been compromised by the disease which prevents her from seeing things in real time and instead ushers in hallucinations). It means spending time with mom even when she does not realize I am there. It means loving on her amazing caregivers at the memory care unit as a way of loving on her.

Loving a person with LBD or any type of memory-based disease is a practice in selflessness and flexibility. It is not a lesson easily learned. Those who do learn it will be better people for it and those that they love will have the freedom to simply be who they are without reservation or judgment. It is a gift, but one we wish others never have to receive.

Chapter 16

There Is No Tired Like Caregiver Tired

Today, as I sit down to write, my husband is sick, so I am relying on caffeine to keep me functioning after a couple of nights of sleeping on the couch. I sleep off and on during the night. I toss and turn and then lay still looking at the ceiling fan rotating above me. Sleeping on the couch is not optimal, but it is an effort to keep me well so that I can care for my parents and my family. It is the life of a caregiver, and it is tiring.

Whether you are a primary or secondary caregiver, the work, worry and toll it takes make for a kind of tired that most people have never experienced before. And while it can feel strategically different at every stage of caring for a person with Lewy body dementia (LBD), it is almost always overwhelming.

I say this to offer you comfort for when you begin to feel this in your bones. You are not less than. You are not a wuss. You are tired just as anyone who walks in your shoes would be.

If someone asks me how I am after rising in the morning, my knee-jerk reaction is to say that I'm tired. But how can one already feel that way just moments after waking? Honestly, the tired I am referring to is not the same as that of people who are sleepy. Instead, the tired I feel is more of a permanent state of mental exhaustion. This is because even when things are running smoothly and I have time to rest and/or sleep, my brain either does not get the memo or refuses to abide by it.

In my opinion, there are five primary stages of fatigue for LBD caregivers:

1 Before the diagnosis tired. For me, this consisted of wearing myself down trying to make my mom's actions make sense.

DOI: 10.4324/9781003656890-18

There were so many things I did not understand. I had never heard of LBD at this point. I did not know what to expect, so every bump in the road felt cataclysmic compared to the normal I was used to.

2 Diagnosis tired. With your loved one's diagnosis in hand, this type of fatigue comes from the mind reeling with what to make of this new course of life. You spend time overthinking how you got here, what you could have done to catch it earlier, how life will change going forward and how you can possibly adapt. These questions tend to run on an endless cycle in your head, with the sheer weight of it all exhausting you. And this is, of course, on top of caring for your loved one who is hurting and experiencing so many changes of their own.

3 Maintenance tired. Once you get your feet under you and start to figure out a little bit of the new normal, the maintenance stage comes with challenges of its own. It is easier in this stage to realize the sheer amount of effort, albeit routine, that goes into helping your loved one each day while also trying to care for yourself. This is also about the same time that you realize how much life you are giving up, thanks to this insidious disease and its devastating effects on the one you love.

4 Progression tired. A healthcare professional once explained to me that the decline in LBD is seldom smooth and continuous. Rather, it can follow a path similar to a rollercoaster with ups, downs and crazy upside-down loops – only it is like being blindfolded so that you cannot see when they are coming. Each stage of the progression of this disease requires a new adjustment to routines, expectations and life in general. The learning curve is steep because there is no set guide for what to expect when you have LBD because the experience is different for everyone.

5 Life tired. For me personally, I find this happens in tandem with most of the above stages. I am a mom of two teenagers, so I am part of the sandwich generation. Those of you who share this stage of life know that caring for your parents and your children at the same time can be rewarding but grueling. There are times when I find myself spread so thin, I realize I am not taking care of myself or being present for those I am caring for.

Recognizing the stages of fatigue is the easy part, believe it or not. Figuring out how to remedy them and implement change is what I find most challenging. Because who has time to analyze such things when you are so tired?

The reality is that your life depends on it.

Read that again.

Your life depends on your willingness to take a timeout for rest and care for yourself. If you think that you're just too tired or don't have the time to do so, consider what will happen to your loved one if you are not around or do not have the capacity to take care of them.

Now do you have time?

It's okay if this shakes you up. It means you now realize the importance of resting and caring for yourself. This is a good thing.

It is important to note that resting looks different for everyone. What works for one may not work for another. Sometimes it takes a trial and error method to figure out what works specifically for you.

For me personally, resting can look like this:

- Praying and spending time with Jesus.
- Talking with a friend who understands what I'm going through.
- Watching a movie or reading a good book.
- Eating a healthy meal.
- Doing a workout.
- Building a Lego set (it is a perfect project for the "fixer" in me).
- Having a good, cathartic cry.
- Sleeping in.

Most of the time, none of these things come to me as naturally as they should. They take intention. Some days I nail it and some days I don't.

But when we take steps to rest and rejuvenate and care for ourselves, we are ensuring we can be there to care for those who depend on and need us most. That is the best gift we can give them.

Chapter 17

Friends and Community Are Lifelines

This journey of caring for someone with Lewy body dementia (LBD) or any type of memory disease can be a lonely one. When you spend much of your time at home caring for your loved one, it can be all too easy for much of your former life to fade into the background.

You know how it goes. You are always in such a hurry at the grocery store that you have no time to visit with the people you run into. You cannot remember the last time you went to dinner with friends. Your smartphone is really the only one who seems to know or understand you.

Humans simply are not made to live in isolation.

At times, your community may look like a memory loss caregiver support group. I urge you to proceed with great discernment when choosing a group to commit your time to. There is one group in particular I joined where many of the caregivers were both helpful and insightful. Yet, one individual tended to rant angrily about her loved one. I know they were likely just distraught over their circumstances, but the negativity with which they dominated the conversation became a hindrance to me (and likely others) getting anything out of the group. Perhaps even more alarming, that negativity took away my peace of mind. I eventually chose to leave the group and find emotional support in close friends. The lesson is to choose wisely when deciding where to put your focus. You are looking for reassurance, not discouragement.

While it is true that your usual outings and social schedule may look drastically different than before the diagnosis of your loved one, there are still ways to spend life-giving time with those

DOI: 10.4324/9781003656890-19

who are not caregivers who can pour into you. Make no mistake about it. This is essential, not optional.

In the beginning stages of my mom's symptoms and diagnosis, most of my interactions with friends were limited strictly to phone calls, and that is okay. Those phone conversations were literal life-lines for me when life became too much, as it often did in that season.

I would call a couple of friends from my Bible study who were kind enough to listen and hold my pain over the phone. A close friend, Nancy, was temporarily living overseas but called me at least once a week to check in. Sometimes I cried. Sometimes I talked about what I was going through. Other times I wanted to talk about anything but what I was going through.

While my situation had not changed after those calls, my spirits had and that was worth its weight in gold.

I eventually got to the point where I was able to do more than just phone calls with friends. As a secondary caregiver, I had the luxury of being able to enjoy an occasional breakfast with a friend before beginning my obligations for the day. I treasured these moments more than words can express. It felt wonderful to sit across the table from a friend who wasn't afraid to share in my pain and grief.

There are friends I am certain God sent me in my low-est moments. They seemed to show up in perfect timing with a thoughtful gift like a coloring book and markers, a cross-stitch set or just a kind note with a sweet treat. These little God winks as I like to call them brought me so much joy. These were the gifts that truly kept giving because every time I used or saw these items, it reinforced how many people cared for me and were pray-ing for me and my parents.

If I was feeling this way as a secondary caregiver, I can only imagine how my dad must have been feeling. In an effort to rem-edy that, there were days I would go visit my parents and care for my mom so that dad could simply get out of the house for a while. On her better days, I would even try taking mom some-where close for lunch so dad could be at home by himself for a bit. He needed time to sort through his feelings just like I did.

I would try to be available to stay with my mom on some Friday mornings at dark thirty so my dad could attend his men's Bible study. The men in this group were and still are such a blessing to him. They listen. They pray. They encourage him. They even visit my mom on occasion. Then they rallied around him when he was diagnosed with prostate cancer amidst my mom's LBD journey.

For those who do not find it possible to visit with friends over the phone or in person, there are still options. Hilarity for Charity (HFC) has some wonderful support programs for caregivers that are online to better accommodate caregivers. I personally participated in one of their mindfulness workshops and got so much out of it. They also offer coloring nights in which you can just log on and color and visit with others. These are just two of their many programs. You can go to www.wearehfc.org for a full listing of online programs and other resources.

Do not underestimate the power of a confidant whether they are a friend or leader. Being able to share with a trusted person such as a pastor or therapist may also provide some relief. Some pastors may do in-home visits if they are aware of your situation, and many therapists now offer online sessions that you can participate in the comfort of your own home.

It is important to note that the need for friends and confidants does not end if you decide to hire professional carers for home or if you move your loved one to memory care. You will still be dealing with all the feels and there will continue to be emergencies that will crop up from time to time.

For example, after we moved my mom into memory care and my dad decided to move out of their home of 30 years, cleaning out the house felt incredibly overwhelming to me. With so much downsizing, there were many items to sell, but first I needed to go through every nook, cranny and couch cushion to ensure my mom had not hidden anything valuable there.

My friend, Nancy, knew how hard this would be for me, so she came to help. She worked alongside me for an entire day to check the pockets of clothes, balled up socks, purses and chest drawers to clean out sticky notes, trash and other things my mom had stashed different places. Nancy never complained once and never turned away when my tears fell. I literally could not have done it without her.

I know beyond a shadow of a doubt I would be utterly lost without my friends. They carried me (and still do) in ways they may never know, but I tried to express my gratitude by sending many of them a handwritten note with this poem that I wrote:

> The people of my village are my heart.
> God gave me them to keep from falling apart.
> They call, they listen, they love, they pray,
> The hold me together at the end of a hard day.
> I know not what the journey ahead will hold,
> But I know the path will be lined by these hearts of gold.
> God, thank you for my village and all they are to me.
> I pray blessings upon blessing for this treasured family.
> By Kimberly Pellicore

Don't go it alone. Find your people, hold them close and don't be afraid to let them carry you when you need it.

Chapter 18

Protecting Your Loved One and Yourself

While the eventual progression of Lewy body dementia (LBD) is largely beyond our control, there are steps we as caregivers can take to mitigate the effects for both our loved ones and ourselves.

For instance, consider dropping your loved one off for a haircut. While inside, your loved one claims they do not know you and that they are there against their will. The hairdresser or barber will likely not know what to believe and it could result in the police being summoned. This situation creates a ripple effect and increases agitation for you and your loved one. But what can you do?

Unfortunately, this situation is one my family is familiar with, minus the police being contacted. My mom was desperate to get her hair done at a hair salon she frequented, but the morning of, she became increasingly agitated and frustrated with my dad who would be driving her there. My dad dropped her off at the front of the store making sure she made it inside okay and then sat outside in the car with his eyes on the front doors. I remember him calling me that morning and telling me he was concerned about what she might say inside and if the staff would believe whatever wild tales she might share. If I remember correctly, there was some follow-up to ensure all was okay as several of the employees noticed mom did not seem herself. We were lucky it did not get more out of hand than that.

The incident served as a reminder that we needed to have tools in place to keep my mom, dad and I safe in the event that she should forget who she was or tell someone she had been taken away from her home against her will (with her version of "home" being her childhood house).

DOI: 10.4324/9781003656890-20

Identification bracelets can be an excellent tool. We did this upon my mom's request. One evening during a lucid moment, when she realized what the disease was doing to her memory, she said one of the worst parts of everything was forgetting her own name. As we talked, I asked if it might help to get her a pretty identification bracelet with her name on it so she could simply look down at it and read her name. She quickly agreed and I bought a beautiful rose gold bracelet engraved with her name, Lewy Body Dementia, and an emergency phone number.

The bracelet was ordered initially to help mom remember her own identity, but it was also effective in providing a source of identification and an emergency number should she become lost or confused when out of our company. While the bracelet proved to be quite helpful, we knew it most likely would not be valid proof of her disease should the police become involved if she got lost. This is why we did keep a signed letter of diagnosis from the doctor on file and easily accessible.

Wallet cards fall into the same category as identification bracelets. They can be helpful but are not always effective for the primary reason that they must be carried to be used as proof. Many patients with dementia do not have the wherewithal to carry a wallet every time they are out. This is because they often misplace it or cannot keep up with it. It may be a safer idea for the accompanying caregiver to carry the wallet card. But, again, this may not serve as conclusive proof for police if they are called.

In my family's experience, documentation from a doctor proved to be the most trusted form of proof of my mom's condition. This should be a letter obtained from your loved one's doctor detailing their diagnosis and mental state. Ideally, it is best to have this documentation in both an electronic and a hard copy that has the signature and contact information of the doctor. This tends to hold more weight in the event that the police are called because it can be verified if need be.

I encourage you to secure these protective measures sooner rather than later. Doing so may not keep a crisis from happening, but it could help facilitate the resolution of it. When dealing with dementia-related memory loss, planning ahead and proactively anticipating situations is always preferred to reacting to a problem you never saw coming.

Chapter 19

The Importance of Elder Law Attorneys

As soon as you receive a diagnosis of dementia for your loved one, it can be wise to make an appointment with an attorney as soon as possible. An elder law attorney may be uniquely suited to help in this area. Find a respected and trusted lawyer who has experience with wills and power of attorney as well as dealing with banks, credit cards and retirement accounts on behalf of someone with a progressive memory disease.

At this point in the journey, a caregiver's biggest challenge may be learning what legalities they need to help their loved one with. In other words, an elder law attorney may be required to guide you in terms of what legal documents need to be updated and/or drafted.

Please take action on these items quickly before your loved one's memory disease progresses to the point that they are not able to make decisions for themselves. Now, go back and read that line one more time because it is that important!

If your loved one does not have a will in place, or even if they already do have one in place, an attorney can help ensure everything is up to date. Not only is it important to ensure that the diagnosed individual has a will that distributes their assets according to their wishes, but it is also essential to make clear their wishes about end-of-life medical treatment through a living will.

A living will can come into play if a person is unconscious and cannot make medical decisions for themselves. This may include decisions such as medication for pain management and the use (or not) of feeding tubes.

Legal counsel also aids in setting up a person's advance directive. This document typically deals with an individual's wishes for

DOI: 10.4324/9781003656890-21

their future health. For example, it can include their preferences regarding tissue and organ donations, feeding when they can no longer tolerate food in its regular form and resuscitation matters.

A DNR (do not resuscitate) document can be put into place by individuals who do not wish to be resuscitated after their heart stops. Word to the wise, if your loved one signed a DNR years ago, they may need to have an updated form completed so that it is accepted by hospitals and care facilities.

It will likely be helpful if your loved one gives legal medical power of attorney to a trusted individual before their disease progresses. This allows the appointed person to carry out the loved one's specific wishes regarding medical care.

While some legal documents can be drafted on your own and then simply notarized, in cases like these and in my opinion, it is generally recommended to have them drafted and approved by an experienced attorney. This can minimize questions regarding the soundness of the process and document.

Fortunately for my mom, she had most of the above already in place well before she was diagnosed. Yet, our experience was still anything from simple.

Unfortunately, when it comes to diseases like Alzheimer's, Lewy body dementia (LBD), or any type of dementia really, there are certain institutions and places that will not be easy to work with regarding the above documents. Banks can be particularly difficult as many require their own power of attorney document rather than choosing to honor a legal one drafted by an attorney.

In addition to trouble with legal documents, there could be some additional bumps in the road you run into when caring for a loved one. These bumps may include, but are not limited to, credit cards and drivers' licenses.

After what we have experienced, I personally think it is easier to deal with closing credit cards after a death rather than during the progression of a debilitating memory disease. This seems ridiculously wrong to me. Whether grieving a loss or dealing with dementia, it should not require an act of God to close a credit card account when a person no longer has the proven mental capacity to use it.

Unfortunately, driver's licenses can pose problems as well. If you choose to let your loved one be responsible for their own driver's license, expect them to lose it and often. One woman told me she solved this problem by providing her husband with a pretend ID (not fake...think kids play) and keeping the real ID in a safe place. Aside from losing their driver's license, another issue can be the expiration of it. Many people assume that once a diagnosed person can no longer safely drive, they do not need their driver's license renewed. I am not saying you should get it renewed. I am not saying that you shouldn't get it renewed. Only you can make this decision but just be aware that an updated ID could still be requested for certain things. I'm looking at you, banks (and my face has captions again).

Lastly, don't forget membership cards. If your loved one has a membership or subscription card for somewhere, you could run into trouble if you try to discontinue or cancel it on your loved one's behalf. An attorney should be able to help you find a way around this type of issue.

This is a lot of information to wade through on top of a caregiver's already full plate. It is for this reason that I recommend enlisting the help of a reputable elder law attorney very early on in the process. They should be able to guide you in terms of what you need to do and when you need to do it. Yes, it will be an expense, but a worthwhile one in my opinion as its purpose is to serve and protect you and your loved one through every stage of this harrowing journey.

Chapter 20

Know What Circumstances Call for Professional Help

Early on in my mom's diagnosis, I sought the counsel of my church's senior pastor, Dr. Burt Palmer. As both a pastor and a volunteer chaplain for the Houston Police Department, he was not new to hard and uncomfortable situations like my own. I explained the burdens I was carrying at the time and how I felt at a loss to best care for my mom.

I distinctly remember him sharing with me that one of the best things I could do in that moment was work with my dad to decide now where we planned to draw the line in the sand for the future in terms of getting my mom professional care. He advised that doing this would help eliminate some of the uncertainty I was feeling about the future and give me the confidence to do what I needed to do when the time finally came.

I shared this conversation with my dad and we both agreed to think on these wise words. As luck would have it, we did not have much time to think about it before the not yet determined line in the sand forced our hand.

My phone rang late one evening and it was my mother, who had not known how to use a phone in weeks. Yet, she was calling from my dad's cell phone. She said dad wasn't feeling well and she just thought I should know. Fortunately, I lived just a few miles away, so I hung up the phone and arrived there in a matter of minutes.

My dad appeared to be running a fever and had the shakes. Despite his assurances otherwise, he also seemed to be somewhat disoriented. He had difficulty summoning enough energy to walk. My sister, her husband and her sweet brother-in-law took him to two different urgent care places while I stayed at home with my

DOI: 10.4324/9781003656890-22

mom, but they could not get him in to be seen. Keep in mind, this was during the height of COVID-19, so the healthcare system was overwhelmed. With no available help at urgent care facilities and his health in mind (he was undergoing radiation for prostate cancer at the time), my sister brought him back home and we called an ambulance.

The medics arrived and began recording his vitals. They had detailed questions about what medicine my dad had taken that evening, what had happened prior and his current health status. At that time, my mom was not fit to answer that information, and I had not been there that day and was at a total loss.

I still remember standing in the den watching my mom trying to contribute what she thought was helpful information (but was not), while the paramedic looked at me with bewilderment and sympathy. The world felt like it was crashing in on me all at once. It was hard to breathe, but I knew I could not afford to lose focus.

We sorted through the situation the best we could, and the paramedics decided it would be best to take my dad to the hospital. We were not allowed to accompany him, so my mom and I stayed behind. I felt helpless watching out the living room window as they loaded my dad into the back of the ambulance and drove away.

Mom sat quietly watching the ambulance drive away with dad in it and then asked me if there was anyone we should call for "that nice man." I didn't think it was possible for my heart to break any more than it already had, but it did in that moment.

I spent the rest of the night trying to calm her down and get her to sleep while trying to keep in touch with my dad via text. It was one of the longest nights of my life. Fortunately, the hospital did not have to keep dad long. He was released mid-morning and my sister and her husband picked him up. He had been diagnosed with a lung infection and sent home with some medication.

After he got home, I stayed for a while with mom and dad to make sure everyone was okay. I wasn't sure what to expect in terms of how mom would react to this new development or if she would even recognize dad. Once the representative from the caregiving company arrived for her shift that morning, I filled her in and then went home to get some much-needed sleep so I could come back and check in a little later that afternoon.

I gave my dad a day or two to regroup before I broached the subject, but I think we both knew it was coming. In the moment dad took an ambulance ride to the hospital and mom was left behind not understanding who he was or why he went away, I knew it was time to start seeking additional help. In my personal opinion, part of my dad's deteriorating health was due to the fact that being a primary caregiver is such an exhausting and never-ending job. With him not there to take care of her, I realized we didn't really have a backup plan that could work for more than a few days at a time.

When I approached dad with my concerns, he admitted he had realized the same. We began to research memory homes in earnest. It simply did not make sense to continue risking his physical and mental health when my mom needed a higher level of care than we could provide. This event was our line in the sand and a catalyst for making plans for my parents' future.

Just the other day, I had a friend come to me whose parent has dementia. She wanted to know how I knew it was time to get my mom additional help. I shared with her what my pastor said and how we were faced with the decision before we were able to clearly identify what it would take before we sought extra help. While it blessedly worked out for us in the end, I am well aware that it could have just as easily gone the other way.

Do not wait to make a decision in the moment you find yourself caught between a rock and a hard place. Evaluate your options now and identify when you will seek out extra help for your loved one, for their sake and yours.

Chapter 21

Home and Respite Care

People have all the feels about home care and respite care for patients with Lewy body dementia (LBD). For many, those feelings are strong and unyielding. Let me be blunt, no matter where you stand on this issue, you are doing a grave disservice to yourself and the caregiving community at large by not accepting that everyone is in a different place on this journey at different times.

It is not wrong to want to care for your loved one at home.
It is not wrong to want to enlist the help of home or respite care.
It is not wrong to want your loved one to receive skilled care in a memory home.
The only thing I would add to each of these scenarios is, "...if it is what is best for your loved one."
If a person is doing what is truly best for their loved one, and it is different than what you have chosen for yours, then so be it. Dementia care is not a one size fits all.

Arriving at the decision to finally do home care for my mom was a journey for me personally. In the beginning, my dad and I felt certain we were not at the point where we needed home care since he lived with mom and my sister and I were minutes away. Was each day perfect? No, it was not. Was our care of her flawless? No, it was not. Were we handling it? We were.

The problem? It was costing us dearly. Dad was scheduling his errands and mental health breaks around when I could be there to sit with mom. Every time dad had a doctor appointment, lunch with a friend or even just a few minutes alone to

DOI: 10.4324/9781003656890-23

himself way from the house, it essentially required a babysitter. The problem was that I was working part-time and also raising two teenagers. Still, we fell into somewhat of a routine and learned to expect the unexpected. With all that both of us were juggling, I'm ashamed to say I never sat still long enough to notice how hard this arrangement was on my dad's health or even my own.

I was constantly tied to my phone in case an emergency call came through from my dad. My body physically reacted every time it rang. My heart rate sped up, my body would tremble and hives seemed to develop instantaneously. If these are the things I experienced as a secondary caregiver, I can only guess how intense things must have felt for my dad.

Because we were "handling" mom's situation on our own, we had not set any real benchmarks for if or when home care would be needed. As life usually does when we are inactive on an issue that needs attention, life decided for us.

Mom's doctors prescribed one of the prescription drugs commonly offered to patients who have LBD. Even though the medication is designed to simply slow down the progression of the disease, I naively thought we would see improvement in some areas. That was not the case. In fact, the first two weeks of taking the medication while her mind and body adjusted were the worst she had experienced to date.

I am sharing some of the lessons my family learned from this journey in hopes that it may help you in your own.

1 The memory of someone with LBD can change on a dime. Just because your loved one knows you now does not mean they will still know you in ten seconds. Plan accordingly and always be prepared to adapt.
2 A loved one wandering or running away due to fear of not knowing where they are or who they are with could result in a call to the authorities by well-meaning bystanders.
3 Unless you have proper documentation to prove that your loved one does indeed have a dementia diagnosis, it is simply your word against theirs which can make it more difficult for a third party to know who to trust.
4 Emergency personnel can only make so many welfare visits for a wandering person before their hand may be forced by local

and state regulations to find more suitable care (a nursing or memory care home) for the individual in question.

For my mom's specific situation, home care became the next logical step. It was something my dad and I originally railed against, but life had other plans. Part-time carers in the home needed to become the new normal because it was the best thing for my mom.

I will pause here to give you a reference of what home care looked like for us. Most days, a person from the home care company spent some time at my parents' during normal business hours (although they offered around the clock care for those who needed it). The majority of these individuals did not have a medical background, but did have experience in caring for people with memory issues. When you compare this with my other chapter about our personal experience with doctors and nurses, you will see that having a medical background does not automatically solve all the problems.

Each day a person would come to the house to help. This entailed light help with small chores, occasionally cooking a meal for my parents, helping to fold laundry, spending time with my mom playing games, walking, doing puzzles or watching television.

For our family, it was never about really needing extra help. It was about needing a third party present who could be a confidant for my mom and a buffer for my dad if she forgot who he was. It was so that someone could still be with mom if dad had an appointment or needed a nap because she kept him up the night before with her hallucinations. This was an invaluable service.

I also know my family was incredibly blessed to be able to afford part-time home care and that not everyone has that same luxury. Still, I do think that these lessons are applicable whether you use a home care company, or you occasionally rely on family and neighbors to help step in when you need a small respite.

Unfortunately, LBD often comes with vivid hallucinations and paranoia or conspiracy theories. We found this to be a constant, so we made sure close family knew to expect it. Friends and family who step in for a regular caregiver may not expect it, causing it to be somewhat of a traumatic experience for them. For this reason, it is important to rely on caregivers that you can resolutely trust. This way, when a wild story emerges such as your loved one telling their regular caregiver that a substitute caregiver is stealing from the home or is taking them on flights to different cities, you can have more confidence this is indeed not the case.

Even though the home care company paid its workers, we made sure to show our appreciation. Whether it was baking some holiday goodies or painting an ornament for them, it was important to us to convey our gratitude to those who helped us in ways they may never quite realize.

One last word about home care companies, be prepared that it can be difficult for these businesses to find and retain people. Unfortunately, this is common throughout memory care centers, nursing homes and home care. When you find an excellent home care representative that your loved one bonds with, make sure that person feels immensely appreciated. We were fortunate to have several of these representatives, with one quickly becoming like family for the love and respect she showed my mom and the support she offered my family. My family still keeps in touch with her to this day.

In my opinion, home care may not be so much for the person with LBD as it is for their caregivers. Professional caregivers offer a buffer and a respite that many family members need to protect their own health and increase their bandwidth for caring for loved ones.

Whether you are a nursing/memory/home care employee or you are simply a caring friend or neighbor, bless you for the ways you support families impacted by memory loss. We could not make this journey without you.

Chapter 22

Making the Move to Memory Care

Not everyone will make the choice to move their loved one to memory care. For some, the issue may be a financial one. Others will tell you it is an issue of honor. For these reasons, moving (or not) a loved one to memory care tends to be a volatile subject. I can understand why this tends to be so.

In this spirit, I will offer the following disclaimer: Unless you are open to moving your loved one to memory care at some point, this chapter may not be for you. No judgment. Feel free to skip to the next chapter.

For those who think moving their family member to memory care could be in the future, the first step is to determine how you will know it is time. The danger in waiting to see how things play out is that without a firm boundary, it becomes all too easy to keep moving the goal line. This leaves you in a state of delayed decision-making that could potentially cost you and your loved one.

My family fell into this camp initially. It seemed too difficult to define a set boundary in which we would know it was time. I think we were looking for a definitive sign rather than setting a benchmark of our own.

For us, the decision to move mom to memory care came when caring for her began to be an issue for my dad. After enduring radiation and fighting prostate cancer, he was understandably tired. He did not have the energy or perseverance that he had just months earlier and it had also earned him a hospital stay. In the meantime, mom's needs were becoming greater. It essentially became an issue of supply and demand. She needed (and deserved) more than we could physically provide.

DOI: 10.4324/9781003656890-24

After coming to that decision, we were fortunate to have a dear home care aid that we discussed this with. Although she knew moving mom to memory care meant she would soon be out of a job, she agreed with us that mom needed more specialized care and dad needed rest to recover from his own health problems.

Once we knew moving her to memory care should be the next step, it was time to look for a potential care center. With hours and hours of research to guide me, I assembled a checklist of questions to present at each home we looked at. I am including many of these points below for your consideration as you do your own research:

Things to verify about the facility itself:

- Name.
- Licensing and certification.
- Number of rooms and beds.
- Security protocol for protecting patients.
- Waiting list for new residents.
- Capacity of facility.

Things to verify about staff:

- Number of memory care staff.
- Staff-to-patient ratio and if this ratio changes overnight or on weekends.
- Type of training staff members receive.
- Frequency of staff training.
- Staff turnover rate (beware this will most likely be high).
- Accreditation of the facility and staff.
- Presence of a certified dementia care manager (CDCM) on-site.
- Presence of staff specifically familiar with Lewy body dementia.

Things to verify about medical care:

- Assistance for patients with incontinence issues.
- Medication protocol.
- Presence of a registered nurse present 24/7.
- Presence of a psychologist (helpful for dispensation of anxiety medications).

- Presence of a resident or visiting physician.
- Ability to bring hospice in house when needed.
- Medical emergency procedure.
- Additional available medical services offered in-house.
- Accepted insurance plans.
- Available *a la carte* care services.

Other things to verify:

- Individual patient assessment and care plan formation.
- Protocol for aggression or bad behavior by patients.
- Dementia techniques utilized.
- Opportunities for patients to get some fresh air.
- Structured activities for patients.
- Patient access to food.
- Pet policy.
- Special seasonal activities for patients.
- Use/availability of music for patients with dementia.
- Exercise program.
- Hairdresser access.
- Patient checkout policy.
- Visitation policy.
- Patient discharge policy.
- Campus security.
- Caregiver/family support group.
- Communication protocol between facility and families.

Things to verify for finances:

- Monthly cost and what is included (may depend on accommodation choices).
- Placement fees.
- Transportation fees.
- Accepted forms of payment.

Feel free to add or subtract from this list as you see fit. Try putting it into an excel spreadsheet and then fill out the fields for each home that you visit. This makes comparisons easier.

My dad's plate was full and overflowing, so my sister and I took over visiting potential care facilities, and then I catalogued the information into a spreadsheet. Once we chose our two favorite facilities, those are the ones my dad went to visit. Then, with our research and input, he made the final decision.

After you have chosen a memory care facility, the next step is to determine how you will execute the move. How advanced the disease is may determine this stage more than any other factor. Some people choose to tell their loved one they are moving. Others take them for a "visit." There is no one-size-fits-all solution here. You need to do what works best for your loved one and family.

Beware that once a decision is made and you are certain it is the right one to make, you may still have periodic doubt. For example, my dad set a date for the move and the week leading up to it was one of the best my mom had in a long time. However, my dad always says that in God's mercy, He let mom have a truly horrible weekend just two days before the move which reminded dad why he made the decision in the first place – because mom needed more care than he was able or qualified to provide.

The last step is knowing what to pack for your loved one to take with them to the home. Keep in mind this is not a typical move. Do not bring things that you are not okay with losing. No matter how careful you are to label everything (and you should), items still tend to walk off because patients forget which room is theirs and what items are theirs. It happens, so plan to be flexible.

Fortunately, the memory care unit we chose offered fully furnished rooms at no extra cost, so we went with that. With mom's memory already gone and her never recognizing her house as home, it would not have made her any more comfortable to bring things from her house. For this reason, we stuck with packing the basics such as:

- Pillow (labeled).
- Seven complete outfits (labeled).
- Ten pairs of underwear (labeled)/or several boxes of disposable diapers if needed.
- Ten pairs of nonslip socks (labeled).
- Two non-hoodie jackets (labeled).

- Five framed pictures (frames best to buy at a dollar store in case they get broken or go missing).
- Two pairs of shoes (labeled).
- Five pairs of pajamas (labeled).
- Three books (if they can still read) (labeled).
- Two blankets (labeled).
- Door/shadow box decorations (labeled).
- Hangers for closet (labeled).
- Two empty bags/purses (labeled).
- Toiletries (but no clippers or sharp objects).

Everything I have included in this chapter is somewhat of a reflection of what was right for my mom and our family. It may not match what is right for yours.

As you approach the milestone of moving your loved one to a memory care center, it is important to make the experience your own. The goal of this chapter is to simply give you a place to start.

Chapter 23

Visiting Memory Care

One of the best tips someone shared with me about visiting memory care is not to have any expectations, because without them, there is no danger of your expectations not being met. In other words, adopting this type of attitude frees us up as family members and friends to meet our loved ones where they are.

It is easier said than done though, I'm afraid. I would be remiss if I didn't tell you it took me a while to let go of my expectations. About 95% of the visits I did have expectations for went up in flames. Most of the time, I had no one to blame but myself.

The hardest visit to the memory care center was my very first visit with mom post move in. The day we moved her in, I stayed for a while, and it went well. The first real visit after that did not. There was a time I questioned if mom was ready to go to a memory care facility simply because she just did not seem as old or late into her diagnosis as other residents. A week after moving her in, I went to see her (they asked us to give them a week to get her acclimated before we visited) and had a major reality check. I am not sure what I expected, but it was definitely not what I got.

My mom was in the activity room with other residents, and she blended in so well I did not even know it was her. That is how much her appearance changed. Mind you, she was perfectly healthy, dressed and well cared for. She just did not look like my mom. I think just not having to keep up the pretense of being fine all the time allowed her to just be true self, which is someone she was used to keeping hidden. I went and sat with her, hoping to have a nice chat. She was angry and what she said did not make sense. She was telling me things that occurred in the past week

DOI: 10.4324/9781003656890-25

(such as plane rides and flooding) that could not have actually happened. I was completely at a loss.

More than a year later, I was discussing this phenomenon with a friend whose mother had been recently diagnosed. My friend was able to define the process beautifully with one word, showtiming. It refers to the ability of an individual with dementia to "put on a show" in which they seem to be holding everything together just fine. In fact, they can be so good at this, there are times in which people may doubt there is anything amiss. However, showtiming is strictly temporary. When a person with dementia is trying desperately not to make mistakes in front of others, they may participate in showtiming. Yet, when they are in the company of people with some of the same struggles, they no longer feel the need to pretend as if all is fine.

Any time you make a visit to the memory care facility, it is critically important to meet your loved one, and others who reside there, where they are. There was one woman my mom befriended who would walk the halls one day and spend the next scooting down the hallways in a defunct crab walk. You never knew for sure which way she would be ambulating each day. There was another gentleman that used to walk laps with my mom and I when she was still able to do so. He often took our hands in his or put his hands on our shoulders while whispering unintelligible words. It was just how he rolled and so we rolled with it too.

Some trips to see my mom were filled with compatible silence in which I simply appreciated that we could peacefully coexist in that time and space. Other trips were quite the opposite in that she wanted no part of me and would send me home. I tried not to take it personally, especially since she never knew who I was.

If you ever babysat for someone growing up, you know the value of bringing a fun activity bag with you. The kids love it because it is something different and the things in that bag are items picked out with them in mind. The same can hold true of visiting your loved one in memory care. You can read a book, play music, sing, brighten up their room with a poster or sweet cards or even decorate their room for an upcoming holiday. I have tried all of these with my mom at one time or another. What is successful once won't always be that way the next time you try it. And an activity your loved one currently hates may soon become their favorite. Bring lots of choices to pick from and be flexible.

I almost always bring her a special treat too, although she never acknowledges that she is excited by it because of the nature of the disease. Still, I will bring her a favorite cold drink and maybe candy or something I have baked. It just helps spread a little proverbial sunshine.

Visiting my mom at memory care has spanned multiple seasons: walking, sitting in the wheelchair and being bedridden. It has not been a linear progression. Nothing about Lewy body dementia (LBD) is linear. It is definitely more like a rollercoaster.

These days, my mom is bedridden and relies on others entirely to help with basic needs. She has a team of amazing helpers from the facility and hospice teams that take care of her daily. These individuals are nothing short of earthly angels.

Depending on a resident's diagnosis and progression, they can be combative at times and pull, push, hit and bite the staff who are trying to help them. While I think most residents do know that they are doing it, I believe it is more of an unconscious defense movement rather than one of malice. However, the result is still the same, which makes being a caregiver challenging to say the very least.

If you visit memory care often enough, you begin to realize this can take a toll on even the best paid workers. It is a physically, mentally and emotionally exhausting job that unfortunately results in an extremely high turnover rate. It bothered me that some of the people who loved my mom best would end up leaving for one reason or another. I wanted to do something to show the staff how much they were loved and appreciated for caring for my mom and hopefully convince them to stay in the process.

I asked a friend whose husband was also in the same memory care facility to band together with me and start a staff appreciation ministry. She has been the best teammate in this endeavor! We take turns bringing a little trinket gift of some sort each month to lift the spirits of staff. For example, National Chocolate Chip Cookie Day is in August, so we brought them chocolate chip cookies and milk. Our monthly gifts are small and our entire budget for 50ish employees is usually $60–$70 a month. The ministry is funded primarily by family members and friends of residents or the occasional volunteer group.

It is amazing the smiles our monthly gifts bring. After all, it is always nice to feel noticed and appreciated. Our hope is that it encourages staff to stay rather than follow the high turnover trend. While I can't speak on behalf of what the employees think about our efforts, I can tell you it brings me great joy and fills my cup to be able to show them that I see and appreciate all the hard work they are putting in day after day.

I find this ministry to be increasingly healing, especially on the days when visits with my mom are brutal. For example, if she is not accepting hugs that day, I can still love on her indirectly by showing my thanks to the people who care for her. In a small way, this ministry is a way for me to give in to my "fixer" tendencies since there is nothing about this disease I can truly fix. The goal is to create smiles and warm fuzzies along the way.

Despite running the memory care staff ministry which fills me up, there are some visits that are harder than others. This you can bank on. Do your best to go with the flow and not put pressure on yourself or your loved one.

No matter what stage of memory loss your loved one is in, I encourage you to visit them...and often. Just because they are cared for by others does not mean they don't need to hear your voice, feel your touch or know that you are there...even if they are unable to put it into words. On the flip side of this, remember that your visits should be lifegiving. If they begin to agitate you or your loved one, it may require change to the type or frequency of visits. The name of the game is flexibility, for the sake of your loved one.

Chapter 24

Anticipatory Grief

It is a strange thing to wholeheartedly miss a person you love and care for deeply when they are sitting right in front of you. Yet, I do it all the time.

I miss the version of my mom before this ruthless disease struck her. I miss the hugs, the laughter, the shopping trips, the movie nights, the girls trips, the card games and at least a million other things that I have grand memories of joyfully doing with her.

As I silently sit with her today, my brain knows this person is my mom, but the woman before me no longer resembles her in appearance nor personality. As she stares blankly into space, I feel that if she had the ability to use words, she would ask who I am and why I am here.

But here we sit, knee to knee on a comfy green couch as she mumbles syllables to herself that I cannot understand. How is it possible to miss my mom when she is so close that I can reach out and hold her hand?

The term is called anticipatory grief. It can be experienced by a caregiver, family or friend who has a loved one enduring a prolonged illness in the months or years before their eventual death.

Knowing that these uncomfortable feelings of loss and grief for an individual who is still living have an actual name made me realize I am not alone in feeling them. I hope this brings you peace as well. There is comfort in knowing others have experienced these same heart-wrenching feelings and have lived to tell us about them.

From a practical standpoint, anticipatory grief can be quite helpful in terms of having sufficient time to research and make

DOI: 10.4324/9781003656890-26

important decisions about the affected person's care both now and in the future.

From an emotional standpoint, anticipatory grief can be viciously cruel because it enables you to mourn the loss of your loved one every day they grow closer to death and then mourn all over again when they finally do pass.

For some, this period from diagnosis to death is a somber but valued opportunity to make amends, spend time together and ultimately make peace with the situation. This is what I sincerely wish for you. Truly. However, this has not been my personal experience. Lewy body dementia (LBD) has now taken so much of my mom that some days she is now agitated by simply my presence because she does not know me, cries because she doesn't understand or recoils from physical touch.

So, what does anticipatory grief look like? I suspect it is different for everyone, but this is how it often looks for me.

- Picking up the phone to text my mom about exciting things happening in the lives of her grandchildren before realizing that while she is still here, she cannot speak, operate a phone, understand how it works or recognize her grandchildren.
- Watching my dad celebrate more than 50 years of marriage with her by bringing my mom a cupcake that he explains away as a "just because" treat so she won't become angered by being told she is married when she has no recollection of those years of memories.
- Wanting to call and ask my mom a million questions about sending my oldest to college and ask her for words of wisdom until I remember that she cannot recall me or the days when I left home for college.
- Lamenting the fact that despite eating well, mom's care team says she is losing weight at a concerning rate which might signal a dramatic decline.
- Watching my daughter shed tears because she would give anything to have her grandmother as her guest at a Mother's Day tea instead of looking at an empty seat.
- Feeling fight or flight kick in when the phone rings in the late overnight hours for fear of a phone call that she has fallen or is sick or is not doing well.

Some of these feelings would be much the same for a person grieving a loved one that passed away suddenly and unexpectedly. However, with anticipatory grief one could experience these same feelings every day for years on end before death as they watch the person they love slowly disappear.

If I had to describe anticipatory grief to someone unfamiliar with the term, I would define it as missing a person you love deeply who is still here but is being worn away daily by disease. It is hard. It comes with tears. And your heart will hurt.

This pain is real and valid and should not be hidden away. But as I keep reminding myself, grief in any form is somewhat of a privilege because it means you were lucky enough to love someone so completely with your whole heart that their absence (whether physical or mental) now takes a piece of yours. There is something truly beautiful about loving another person so fully and with that kind of abandonment.

During my 47 years on this earth, I have been blessed to be loved by my mom. This, I have no doubt, is one of my greatest blessings.

On the days when life feels particularly heavy or the tears flow freely with grief, I do not scold myself for feeling this way. It is a part of my personal journey to healing. What I am working on is not letting grief erase all the amazing joys loving my mom has given me.

It is fun to recall the sweet memories that remind me of her. Mom introduced me to the deliciousness that is peanut butter and pickle sandwiches (don't knock it until you try it). She taught me the importance of the quest to find the perfect purse for each season. She made ginger molasses cookies in a way that no one has been able to successfully replicate. She taught me how to laugh until I cried over card games like Rummy and Liverpool. She showed me what a mom is supposed to be and encouraged me in my own journey in that role. She gave me my love of words. She loved and supported me unconditionally.

This is the mom I will remember. I know she is still there somewhere in the woman that sits before me now. Just as I know she struggles to remember me, I must try to remember the real her and hold those memories close.

Chapter 25

Tomorrow Is Not Guaranteed

For everyone, it is a given that tomorrow is not guaranteed. As caregivers, we have seen too much, grieved difficult circumstances and mourned too much loss to believe any different. While in some ways, I think it can be healthy to acknowledge that we all have an expiration date from the time we enter this world as a baby, and there are other ways in which it can mess with our brains.

Especially when in the thick of emergency phone calls, crisis situations and the rigor of caring for a loved one with Lewy body dementia (LBD), the brain has what I have heard referred to as having too many tabs open. As caregivers, our brains are trying to process the challenges of yesterday, making it through today and sometimes anticipating what we might could expect the next day. That vicious cycle of thinking and rethinking can make my brain feel tired and that is when I realize with terror that my own brain is starting to slip.

In visiting with fellow caregivers for people with memory disease, I have found it is not unusual for caregivers to notice a change in their own cognitive abilities because of the emotional and mental weight they carry every single day. And because of my exposure to my mom's diagnosis, I start to wonder if I could be "getting it" too. While memory diseases like LBD are not considered to be at all contagious, if your parent or grandparent has the disease, it is somewhat natural to wonder if you are next.

I have a friend who is in much the same boat as I, and we speak frequently about the ways our brains betray us. Either it is a name we cannot remember, an ingredient we forgot to put in dinner or the place we put the birthday card we need to mail out

DOI: 10.4324/9781003656890-27

next week. We both do it and it gives me peace to know her brain taps out sometimes too. We are not losing it. We are simply doing too much all. the. time.

As caregivers, we are doing so many things – especially those of us in the sandwich generation where we care for parents and children at the same time. Our brains are only designed to handle so much. One of the best ways to remedy this is to take better care of ourselves.

I know. "When on earth am I supposed to do that?" you say. I get it. But I also know that if you do not voluntarily make time to care for yourself, your body will demand it from you. Ask me how I know.

I am just now, after five years, starting to put myself back together again, and I am continually astonished at how far I let my health and well-being get away from me.

In this season, I am taking the phrase "Tomorrow is not guaranteed" and changing how I think about it. Instead of focusing on all the negatives the phrase could imply about my mother and even myself, I am choosing to think about it differently. What would my mom tell me to do if she could truly see me now?

I feel in my heart that I know exactly what she would say.

"That trip you have always wanted to take? Do it now while you can."

"That book you have always wanted to write? Start it now."

"That small business you have dreamed of building? Stop dreaming and do it."

"That nudge to tell your family and friends how much they mean to you? Listen to it."

"The dishes in the sink when your daughter asks you to spend time with her? Leave them."

"The house you should clean when you have time to take a nap? Sleep."

"The holidays you decorate and work yourself into a frenzy for? Remember it is the people that make it special."

I feel like every statement above and dozens more like it would be her way of telling me that after a season in which I stopped living life, it is high time to begin again and do so in her honor. There will always be days in which anticipatory grief will sneak up on me and overtake me. That is grief doing what grief does. No judgment. But living exclusively in grief every single day is not helping my mom, and it is not helping me.

Make today the day you realize the lessons your loved one is teaching you as they walk through this terrible disease. Then learn from them and make your loved one proud.

Chapter 26

You Will Not Be the Same Person

When I look back now on the person I was before my mom's struggle and diagnosis with Lewy body dementia (LBD), I scarcely recognize myself but in a mostly good way.

The woman I see in hindsight was wrapped up in her own life. She was a good person, but maybe a little too self-focused at times and tended to take things for granted. I remember distinctly coming home from a girl's shopping trip a few months before the unmistakable symptoms of the disease set in. My mom, teenage daughter and I were coming home from the mall, and I was complaining endlessly about some trivial inconvenience.

What I would give to have that car ride home back again. I would like to think my current self would pause talking long enough to revel in the fact I was blessed to be spending this time with some incredible women in my life. I would like to think I would do less talking and more listening. And I would wish for that car ride to go on forever so I could memorize every moment.

In the end, I am not the same person I was before my mom's diagnosis. Over the last several years, I have come to the conclusion that it is mostly for the better. And I think it would be a mistake not to acknowledge that this growth came out of much turmoil and angst. It was not just an afternoon epiphany.

Looking back, I can see three stages to my transformation:

1 Acceptance.
2 Fight or flight.
3 Reckoning.

DOI: 10.4324/9781003656890-28

From the moment our family noticed something was a little off for mom, I felt certain it would turn out to be as simple as a vitamin deficiency. After all, mixing up a few dates and forgetting a couple of small things was not the end of the world. At this point, there were no earthshattering symptoms present. But after quarantining and social distancing during the pandemic, a stunning collapse in mom's cognitive abilities developed as well as her ability to recognize her family or even the year.

Acceptance

Getting the right doctor visits lined up with a primary doctor, a neurologist and a memory testing facility for a diagnosis then led to MRIs and prescriptions to hopefully temper the LBD as well as the anxiety my mom was experiencing. While I was able to accept that this was indeed happening and that things would be forever different going forward, do not confuse my acceptance of her diagnosis with the embracement of it. Those are two entirely different things.

Fight or Flight

Then came the fight or flight stage. This was by far the most traumatic stage for me, but I also think it cleared the path for eventual transformation. Fight or flight became a moment-to-moment way of life for me characterized by frantic phone calls from my mother wanting to know who the man in her house was (my dad), calls to come meet my parents at the curbside grocery pickup because mom had suddenly forgotten who dad was and would not get back in the car, calls from mom to come get her because she believed someone kidnapped her, calls from mom when she was overcome with fears and tears and calls from dad to let us know mom had called the police because she recognized no one.

My heart quickens and I feel the beginnings of hives breaking out on my skin just rewriting this barebones summary of that season. It was an awful couple of years in which there seemed to be no rest. Emergency mode reigned all the time. There was no time to think, only to do. There was no thriving; there was just surviving. It consumed me in ways I am not proud of. It was ridiculously hard on my health and my family, and the effects still linger today.

When it became apparent that professional caregivers needed to be part of the equation for the sake of both of my parents and myself, we thought enlisting their help would provide some much-needed relief. And while there were periods of respite, they were not common or predictable. This left my dad exhausted and myself feeling the effects of flight or flight again. We continued on this way for over a year before it became incredibly apparent that mom needed full-time care for a better quality of life.

It broke my family to move mom to a local memory care home, but we all knew beyond a shadow of a doubt, it was the right thing to do for both my mom and my dad.

Now, almost two years post move in, things have become by and large more routine for mom and us. There are still hiccups and hospital visits and trauma along the way, but it is no longer daily. The fight or flight from mom's situation has now mostly settled, but more often than not, I still feel like my body is stuck in that mode. It is like the switch is stuck and I cannot flip it off.

Reckoning

My heart is still broken. My health is not what it should be. But my mom is safe and my dad's health is improving.

For the first time, I am beginning to realize that for the last five years, I have lived and breathed my mom's diagnosis, although I'm not entirely sure that was actually a choice. With her now settled and well cared for, I have the bandwidth to survey the collateral damage. It is far vaster than I could have ever imagined – mentally, physically and emotionally.

But life must go on. And this involves reckoning because change only happens when we move forward.

In this leg of the journey, I am noticing new things about the person I have become. I am trying to focus on my parents and my own family. I work hard to stay connected to friends whose love and support have carried me the last few years. I truly value them in a way I did not before and make sure they know I am there for them too, although I often still feel I fall short because of all I am balancing. I push myself to do hard and uncomfortable things like writing this book now, because the future is not guaranteed. I do my best to remain mindful that the world is not mine to carry or control.

Because I am not the same person I was before this journey started, I am struggling to find which hobbies I now enjoy. I am studying how to relax. I am trying to let my body rest when it signals that it needs it. I am learning what it is to be a daughter with a mom who is still physically here but mentally is not. I am discovering how to be a mother with one child nine hours away in college and another headed to college soon. I am refocusing on my mental and physical health. And mostly, at the end of the day, I continue to put one foot in front of the other. I am trusting that the work I am putting in will be worth it. This is what my mom would want for me.

Remember, the journey as a primary or secondary caregiver of a patient with LBD is a haggard one filled with mountains and valleys. While you may need to mourn the life you thought you would have compared to the one you will have at the end of this journey, take heart in knowing that the journey can give way to hope and new beginnings.

Chapter 27

When the End Is Near

Wednesday of last week, I found out that despite the memory care home's best efforts, my mom's weight fell by eight pounds. The knowledge that her weight is continuing to drop has felt like a rock sitting in my stomach that I carry with me everywhere I go. There's no getting rid of it. Distraction is only temporary. The rock feels like it's here to stay.

In the meantime, we attended a funeral for a dear friend of my dad's who has been a godsend to him throughout my mom's journey with dementia. He was a wonderful man who passed away unexpectedly and at a relatively young age. As my dad and I honored this man whom we both respected by attending his funeral, I think the realization that we could be doing this soon for my mom was present too.

Today, my dad visited mom and found out her weight continues to go down even since last week. I hear the pain he is feeling for her as she battles the evils of dementia almost more clearly than the words he actually says. It drifts through the phone and fights for a space in my already broken heart and a place on my shoulders.

Some days it just feels like the loss is piling up if I am being honest.

Since the day my mom was diagnosed, I've known the end was coming. And really, that shouldn't be news for any of us. From the day we are born into this world, our lives have an expiration date. However, I think having a diagnosis that comes with a more definitive timeline can make a person (and the people around them) more cognizant of it.

DOI: 10.4324/9781003656890-29

I say this not out of morbidity, but to hopefully bring you a sense of relief. We will all pass one day and there is nothing that I, you or anybody else can do to keep that from happening. There is some freedom in that for me, to know that it is beyond my control and not something I am responsible for. As a child of God, there is also the knowledge that the Father puts us here for a reason but when our time on Earth is done, He is not done with us. He will heal us completely when we enter Heaven's gates, and we will experience a fuller life there than we have ever known here on Earth.

During mom's journey, I've met some individuals who believe that if a caregiver's faith is strong enough, it will keep the sorrow from coming. I do not believe this to be true at all.

Even Jesus felt sorrow at the passing of his good friend, Lazarus (John 11:35). As caregivers and loved ones of a person with dementia, God doesn't expect us to endure that which we are without feeling sorrow either. The Christian Walk is not a journey without hardship. In fact, Jesus promises us that trouble will be a part of it (John 16:33). Even so, He kindly walks through it with us, never leaving our side (Psalm 147:3).

Despite walking with Jesus, this path of sorrow is not outwardly pretty. I have faith Jesus will work all things for good in the lives of those who believe, but He never promised me easy street this side of Heaven. So, there are days where I camp out in the valley of self-pity, tears and heartbreak which can look a lot like staying in my pajamas, napping and avoiding life beyond the walls of my home. Other days, it can look similar to what it did before my mom's diagnosis, a hint of a smile and a lift in my step, until I remember.

Some people tend to see a return to sadness after experiencing a brief moment of joy as a failure in finding hope. I don't. Grieving, especially anticipatory grieving, is a rollercoaster of feelings and emotions. There will be highs and lows, twists and turns. It is simply the nature of the journey. A couple of light-hearted days do not mean grief won't strike again and a week of sadness does not mean joy and hope are beyond you.

There have been days where it has been far too easy to sink into a deep hole of self-pity and sadness at what my mom is enduring and how it has changed almost every facet of my family's lives.

While it is okay to feel the feels for a time, it cannot be where you or I stay. Cry. Be angry. Embrace pity. But then climb out of the hole. If it is too deep to make it out on your own, call on Jesus.

God doesn't want us to stick our heads in the sand and pretend everything is okay because it is what good Christians do. No... just no. He wants you to know that even amidst the journey you are on, He is there for you and will sustain you when your own strength and stamina fall short. He brings the sunshine and the joy so that you can continue to endure the sorrow without being decimated by it.

But what about our loved ones that we are either still actively caring for or whom we visit in a memory care home? Do you ever wonder how an individual who is not of sound mind and who cannot form clear words communicates with Jesus? It is something I speculate on frequently.

My visits with mom at the memory care unit are different than I once pictured. Before she broke her hip, she walked almost constantly during my visits speaking a blend of vowels and consonants that did not compute. On the rare occasion I could get her to sit and rest with me on one of the home's comfy couches, she occasionally let me hold her hand while she slept. Sometimes we walked together, and sometimes she didn't know me and asked me to leave.

Now, visits are even more different. My mom remains mostly in the hospital bed in her room as her broken hip is still healing and her core muscles (or lack thereof) do not allow her to sit up anymore. While she is not blind, she does not see me and hallucinates constantly. She sleeps a lot, does not like to be hugged and sometimes still motions for me to leave.

It has become increasingly important to me that my mom knows she is loved on a daily basis. It does not matter to me whether she feels loved by my dad, me, a staff member, a fellow resident, the registered nurse or hospice as long as she knows she is loved. Somehow, I feel like that could be significant in healing the sane part of her that is trapped somewhere inside.

Before I got out of my car to go in the home on a previous visit, I prayed God would help me see evidence of this. It was a suggestion my husband had given me and one I thought had merit. That day at the home, I spoke to three very busy staff who all paused to share something good about mom with me – without me asking. I was even fortunate enough to see mom laugh joyfully in her sleep. God's hand was everywhere.

The image of her laughing in her sleep has stayed with me as do the moments when she sincerely smiles in unintelligible conversation with someone I cannot see. From the outside, these could easily be explained as hallucinations, but there is a part of me that thinks Heaven may already be connecting to her soul in a manner I am not privy to. At the end of the day, if whatever these exchanges are bring her some sense of happiness and relief, then I will call them blessings and be thankful.

I do not know how many days I have left with mom, but I sense they are dwindling. There is no way to adequately prepare for the loss of someone you love because our hearts were never meant to be broken. So, for now, in between sleepless nights and a few tears, I am resolving to continue visit my mom often and pray for her constantly. This is the extent to which things are under my control. God has the rest.

Chapter 28

Life Is Meant to Be Lived

The days have long since passed when my mom and I could have a real conversation of any kind. However, I do have a strong memory of a sweet conversation we shared during one of our visits at the memory care home, and I hold it close.

I had come to see mom for one of our usual visits but was more than a little apprehensive as our most recent time together had not gone well. It ended with her confusing me with someone else and requesting that I go home.

On this new day, mom still did not know me but apparently recognized me as friendly. We didn't really talk to one another because she seldom was able to engage in conversation. She did, however, allow me to walk with her down the hallways of the home. I even got a tentative smile. It felt like winning the lottery.

After almost 20 minutes of walking, mom motioned to a corner sitting area furnished with a velvet green couch, two sitting chairs and a television. We sat together in a comfortable silence on the couch. The longer we stayed there, the more she leaned toward the arm of the sofa and eventually dozed off. I watched her sleep peacefully and was overjoyed to hear a small laugh escape from what must have been a wonderful vision or dream.

Though holding hands was not something she was usually receptive to, since she was asleep, I gently placed my hand over hers. Surprisingly, she felt the light pressure and reacted by turning her hand over to hold mine. Tears formed in the corners of my eyes. Grateful did not even begin to cover it.

We stayed like that for more than an hour. I was in no hurry to move for fear I would wake her, and all her peace and relaxation would vanish. I turned to speak with another patient who

DOI: 10.4324/9781003656890-30

often followed mom and I around. We spoke for only a minute or two. When I eventually turned my gaze back to my mom, she was staring at me.

Although she was lying in much the same position, her head was turned toward me, her eyes were open and her gaze piercing. I held my breath not knowing what version of my mom would emerge from her nap.

My mom sat up and linked one of her arms through mine (this on its own was nothing short of a miracle). With her other arm, she gently patted my shoulder and softly said with a smile, "Kim, promise me that when you can do something fun, you will." Before I could respond, she dozed off again and the moment was gone.

There is a part of me that firmly believes she fought like hell to be able to share that sentiment with me. She fought the hallucinations, the memory loss and the cognitive challenges of forming a thought all to leave me with this one piece of sage advice.

Whether it was a moment of lucidity or a complete fluke, my mom's words went straight to my heart. That she would fight so hard just to share those words with me made me tear up. I knew what it must have cost her. I also knew that my response would forever be yes.

I promised myself then and there that if I had a chance to take a trip, I would. If I had a chance to do work or do something silly, I would choose silly. If I could do something that brought me joy, I would be all in.

The problem is, I subconsciously categorized these as big things like vacations and special events (things I do not do nearly as often as I should). These absolutely are important for mental health, but sometimes I wonder if she meant to incorporate fun in everyday moments. After all, joyful little moments patchworked together over the years is evidence of a life of joy.

If I am completely honest, I haven't had much, if any, fun since mom was diagnosed and my world changed in really big and long-lasting ways. It is like I don't know how to do it anymore. Every celebration is one I wish she were there for like her grandkids' high school graduations, homecoming dances, college ring ceremonies, holidays and so much more. Her absence seems to suck up some of the joy that those special times bring.

Yet, I cannot help but think this is not what my mom would want for me. This is not what I want for me. I made her a promise that I want to keep.

I have been pondering what this looks like practically when I came across these words by author Ann Voskamp in an Instagram post, "Life is not an emergency. Life is a gift."

And, so I begin. I am finding one of the areas I am lacking in is savoring the little moments (Side Note: For more on this topic, I highly recommend *Soul Care* by Debra Fileta). Fun is not limited to parties and confetti and wild amusement park rides. Fun can also take the form of savoring the moment by:

- Watching a favorite movie with your phone put away.
- Baking homemade cinnamon rolls.
- Crafting.
- Working out.
- Going to lunch with dear friends.
- Reading a book that you don't want to put down.

My mom would hate what this disease has stolen from her. Possibly the only thing she might hate more is what I am also letting it steal from me. It is possible to hold both grief and joy in the same season.

As it turns out, the fun my mom asked me to have is something I have to practice in order to make it come more naturally. Every day is a new opportunity to start anew. Some days I get it right. Some days I fail miserably. But even on the days I fail, I don't really, because if I fail, it also means I tried.

Chapter 29

Finding the Way through Loss

I have heard it said before that losing someone to a memory disease day by day can feel like death by papercuts. I find that statement to be on point. The experience is ongoing. It is painful. It wears you down. Which begs the question, how can anyone survive it?

For years now, my mom has been dealing with late-stage Lewy body dementia (LBD) which seemed to steal her peace and memory suddenly amidst the isolation of the pandemic. There was no season of adjustment or easing into things because it all happened in what felt like the blink of an eye. Normal disappeared and is never coming back again.

When I reflect on the mountains and valleys of the journey thus far, I marvel that I am still here. The lack of sleep, constant worry, worn-down immune system and feeling my heart break into pieces adds up and has real consequences.

The experience has not left me unscathed. Several health issues have popped up that are due largely due to me not taking proper care of myself while reeling from my mom's diagnosis. Some days have been so incredibly difficult that I thought they might best me, but God.

The reason I am still here is God. It is nothing I have done. He gives me breath each morning and is my strength for another day. He is what gets me through. My faith in Jesus is my lifeline.

I marvel at biblical stories like Moses parting the Red Sea. I once focused solely on the miracle. I looked at that example and wanted God to move in that way for my mom, my family and myself. I wanted a grand miracle in which God would sweep

DOI: 10.4324/9781003656890-31

away the dementia just like He swept away the waters of the Red Sea. Could He do it if He wanted to? I absolutely believe so. Does that mean He is going to? No.

Here is the thing. Sometimes I tend to focus on the miracle and not the problems that lead up to it. The Israelites were slaves in Egypt for years and endured incredibly difficult circumstances because of it. Think of their joy when God sent Moses to liberate them from that slavery.

Now, think of how the Israelites must have felt when their trek out of Egypt left them trapped between the waters of the Red Sea and Pharaoh's army bearing down on them. In Exodus 14:11, the Israelites ask Moses, "Was it because there were no graves in Egypt that you brought us to the desert to die? What have you done to us by bringing us out of Egypt?" I think the Israelites were beginning to think God freed them just to die by drowning or at the hands of Pharoah's army. I might have initially wondered the same.

Yet Moses's response to their doubts in Exodus 14:13 is this, "Do not be afraid. Stand firm and you will see the deliverance the Lord will bring you today." Then several verses later in Exodus 14:21, God parted the waters so the Israelites could make their way safely through and escape the army.

There are times when I think of this miracle through the lens of my mom's story. For years, I have watched her struggle with this diagnosis and disease. I have seen all that it has taken from her and our family. Why won't God step in and take the disease away and rescue us right now?

The real answer is I don't know.

So why do I continue to believe my hope rests in Jesus? Because I am studying the Bible and getting to know the character of God. Jeremiah 29:11 tells us He does not wish to harm us, but to give us a hope and future. At no point does He ever say our earthly lives will be smooth sailing. In fact, He says just the opposite in John 16:33, "In this world you will have trouble. But take heart! I have overcome the world."

Knowing these things does not keep me from struggling. There is still anger, sadness and grief. But it does give me hope that there is more to life, both on this earth and in Heaven.

In Isaiah 43:2, the writer shares the Lord's words,

When you pass through the waters, I will be with you; and when you pass through the rivers, they will not sweep over you. When you walk through the fire, you will not be burned; the flames will not set you ablaze.

The problems of life will always be a part of our stories because of our fallen world. Yet, Isaiah 26:3 promises God will give us a perfect peace to keep our problems from overcoming us *if* we are steadfast in keeping our eyes on Him. Even when we don't understand our circumstances and what is happening, God does and we can trust Him with them.

When it comes to my mom's condition specifically, I cling to Hebrews 11:1 which says, "Now faith is confidence in what we hope for and assurance about what we do not see." Although I still see the outer shell of my mom who cannot see or carry on conversation, I believe she already has one foot in Heaven. I think Jesus is already caring for her in ways that I cannot see. Why? Because I know the character of God.

Last week, it became more than knowing, it became hearing. I visited mom at memory care and sat by her bed hearing her utter sounds that did not make recognizable words. Other than that, she was silent for the duration of my visit and, as always, very much in the private world her brain has created. As I was leaving, I leaned in, kissed her head and whispered goodbye. She showed no recognition of my presence or of my words, but as I pulled away she clearly enunciated the word "Jesus." It was just once and no other words or sounds followed it, but I heard it. We had not been talking about Him and He is not someone my mom has mentioned in a couple of years. But there it was, along with an unexplainable peace that immediately filled her room. He was there!

When Moses was in exile, God was still with him. When Ruth had no one to care for her, God was still with her. When David was on the run from King Saul, God was still with him. When Paul was in prison, God was still with him. When Peter denied Jesus three times, God was still with him. In each scenario, the problematic part of the person's story was in play while God was walking with them. The truth is, God had never been apart from them.

God is still with my mom. He is still with me. I don't understand what He is doing, but I believe Him when He says in Isaiah 43:19, "See, I am doing a new thing! Now it springs up; do you not perceive it? I am making a way in the wilderness and streams in the wasteland."

This is forever my hope and stay.

Chapter 30

Epilogue

Writing this book has been a journey in duality. It has been a beautiful and uplifting thing to be able to put words to a page that will hopefully help another caregiver navigate their own Lewy body dementia (LBD) experience without feeling so alone. At the same time, my mom still resides in memory care and her circumstances remain largely unchanged outside of a continued general decline. Reconciling these two experiences has become challenging at times.

It is a profound thing to watch the world around you keep moving at a breakneck pace while your own has come to a grinding halt. I find it impossible to be fully a part of either side. I live somewhere in the in between and this is what life looks like today.

My mom has been in memory care for more than three years and has struggled with visible signs of the disease for six. She is bedridden, cannot care for herself, cannot participate in a conversation and does not have the ability to see her environment or the people in it (thanks to false projections of the brain associated with this disease). I visit her often, but she never reveals any flicker of awareness that I am present. The same is true of my dad's visits to see her. We frequently bring her a favorite drink or treat intended to brighten her day, and although she is not able to communicate it, I do believe it brings her some degree of joy. I long for her deeply, even while she is still here. It is not uncommon for me to pick up the phone to call her before remembering that she will not pick up. My heart still aches, and the tears still come.

My life as a sandwich caregiver remains in flux. Although my dad ultimately decided to move out of his home of more than

DOI: 10.4324/9781003656890-32

30 years, he remains nearby and a regular part of my family's lives. My oldest child is nearing the finish line of his college career, and my youngest will soon graduate high school. Although they both largely take care of themselves, I still immensely enjoy spending time with them and am still needed. Sometimes I wonder if their memories of me during the last six years will be of the mom who supported and loved them dearly or the crazed sandwich generation caregiver trying to wrangle the wild rollercoaster that is LBD. My guess is that their recollections will be somewhere in between, with the acknowledgment that I was always doing the best I could. Or at least that is my hope.

As for me, when I'm not working or doing all the things a wife, mom, daughter and secondary caregiver do, my favorite indulgence is relaxing in my recliner and escaping into the pages or movies of *Harry Potter*. I am working out more and am practicing the art of savoring the moment. I do my best to practice what I preach in terms of taking care of myself, but I am an imperfect work in progress. Some days I get it right. Some days I don't. But I never stop trying.

My sincerest wish is that this book will raise awareness of LBD and be a helpful resource for those walking the caregiving journey with a loved one with memory loss. I believe many of the lessons I have learned and shared in these pages are helpful to caregivers and friends who want to honor loved ones with their interactions.

I am beyond thankful you chose to spend your valuable time with me in the pages of this book. Thank you for letting me share my mother's story and my heart. I am abundantly grateful and yet – no one's life has changed simply because you read this book. The steps you take after reading will determine its impact, whether they be in caregiving or advocacy.

Keep going. I am cheering you on, friend.

For Product Safety Concerns and Information please contact our EU
representative GPSR@taylorandfrancis.com
Taylor & Francis Verlag GmbH, Kaufingerstraße 24, 80331 München, Germany